Psychedelics

A POCKET PRIMER

WRITTEN BY
MATTHA BUSBY

EDITED BY
FLORENCE WARD

Psychedelics: A pocket primer
First edition

Published in 2025 by
Hoxton Mini Press, London
Copyright © Hoxton Mini Press
2025. All rights reserved.

Text by Mattha Busby
Edited by Florence Ward
Production design and additional
artwork by Dom Grant
Series design by Tom Etherington
Cover illustration by Lan Truong
Proofreading by Zoë Jellicoe

The right of Mattha Busby to be
identified as the creator of this
Work has been asserted under the
Copyright, Designs and Patents
Act 1988.

Thank you to all of the individuals
and institutions who have provided
images and arranged permissions.
While every effort has been made to
trace the present copyright holders
we apologise in advance for any
unintentional omission or error,
and would be pleased to insert the
appropriate acknowledgement in
any subsequent edition.

A CIP catalogue record for this
book is available from the
British Library.

ISBN: 978-1-914314-86-5

Printed and bound by Ozgraf, Poland

Manufacturer: Hoxton Mini Press,
104 Northside Studios, 16-29
Andrews Road, London, E8 4QF
www.hoxtonminipress.com

Represented by: Authorised Rep
Compliance Ltd., Ground Floor,
71 Lower Baggot Street, Dublin,
D02 P593, Ireland
www.arccompliance.com

Hoxton Mini Press is an envi-
ronmentally conscious publisher,
committed to offsetting our carbon
footprint. This book is 100 per cent
carbon compensated, with offset
purchased from Stand For Trees.

Every time you order from our
website, we plant a tree:
www.hoxtonminipress.com

FSC
www.fsc.org

MIX
Paper | Supporting
responsible forestry
FSC® C163799

Introduction:
Why should we care about
psychedelics?

Imagine you're living with depression or anxiety, and instead of the usual pharmaceuticals, your doctor prescribes you a trip with psilocybin – the psychedelic compound found in magic mushrooms. You visit a clinic where, under professional supervision, you embark on a guided journey into non-ordinary consciousness. The experience is intense, mystical and – quite possibly – profoundly healing. In the weeks that follow, with the help of therapy, you find the burden of your mental health struggles lifting.

This isn't science fiction: it's a vision psychedelic advocates believe is just a few years away. In some parts of the world, like in the US state of Oregon, guided mushroom journeys are already legal. MDMA-assisted therapy has been approved in Australia and there is a limited access scheme in Canada. Psychedelic start-up companies are investing more and more money into research, and studies increasingly attract public funding. After all, they have the potential to revolutionise not only mental health treatment, but also the way we understand consciousness itself.

This is old news for the communities that have long histories of psychedelic use. Mind-altering plants, including some of those that are popular today, have been treated with sacramental reverence and used for physical and spiritual healing purposes over millennia. Beyond their therapeutic uses, psychedelics also deliver transcendental experiences that can open spiritual doors, connecting us more deeply to each other, nature and even God. A wider acceptance of psychedelics might change not just mental health care, but also our cultural attitudes toward healing, personal growth and death.

As with any paradigm shift, there are uncertainties. We still have much to learn about the long-term effects of psychedelics and how to minimise the risk of experiences that can destabilise people. The Wild West nature of the current grey market industry has also attracted some unsavoury characters, and the rapid growth of the psychedelic industry raises ethical questions. Will these treatments be accessible only to those who can afford expensive clinic visits? How do we ensure these experiences are safe, especially when commercial interests are at play? And how do we honour the Indigenous communities who have long used these substances in their spiritual practices, without simply appropriating their knowledge? Balancing the promise of psychedelics with a cautious, informed approach is critical.

This book is intended to take you on a trip of your own, through the history of these extraordinary drugs up to the present day. With psychedelics teetering on the brink of mainstream acceptance, we'll take a sober look at what they promise, sorting the hype from the hysteria and the fact from fiction.

A little taster
of the key drugs

Before we start, here is a brief introduction to some of the key psychedelic compounds, and the drugs and plants in which they can be found.

PSILOCYBIN

Fungi containing psilocybin grow worldwide and are commonly referred to as magic mushrooms, or 'shrooms'. Used historically by Indigenous people in Mexico, Lesotho and elsewhere, psilocybin is currently being studied as a potential therapy for depression.

MESCALINE

Found in peyote and San Pedro cacti, mescaline was the first psychedelic to be isolated in the lab. It brings about intense nausea, euphoria and deep introspection. Trips are lengthy (up to 12 hours) and characterised by vivid colours and altered sensory experiences.

DIMETHYLTRYPTAMINE (DMT)

A naturally occurring psychedelic found in many plants and animals, with a structure closely resembling happiness hormone serotonin, DMT induces colourful visions. It is often characterised by feelings of breaking through to other dimensions and even encountering entities. Trips are very short, typically lasting no longer than 15 minutes.

IBOGAINE

Derived from the root bark of the iboga plant (native to Gabon), ibogaine has also been heralded for its potential in treating addiction. Perhaps the most powerful of all psychedelics, journeys with ibogaine are sometimes compared with summiting Mount Everest due to the physical and mental intensity of the experience. Users are often treated to fly-on-the-wall-style trauma-processing biopics of their lives.

5-MEO-DMT

Found within the glands of the Sonoran desert toad (the smokable secretions of which are known simply as 'bufo'), 5-MeO-DMT is very different from its cousin, DMT. With trips also lasting about 15 minutes, users can experience a powerful sense of unity, non-dual consciousness or oneness, and clinical studies investigating its effects are ongoing. The visuals are often subtler than DMT, with more focus on the internal experience and ego dissolution. The molecule can also be synthetically produced in a lab.

AYAHUASCA

A psychoactive tea brewed from a shrub containing DMT, ayahuasca is traditionally a ceremonial drug, used by Indigenous populations across South America. It can cause intense euphoria, otherworldly visions and a host of mind-altering effects (plus puking) over nine hours, depending on the dose.

PEYOTE

A stubby cactus containing the active compound mescaline, peyote is traditionally used by Indigenous peoples in the southwestern US and northern Mexico as a sacrament to induce visionary states, promote spiritual insight and treat ailments.

SAN PEDRO

A taller cactus also containing mescaline, San Pedro is used primarily in the Andes, where it grows abundantly in Peru, Ecuador and Bolivia. It is consumed for much the same purposes as peyote, though by different Indigenous groups.

LSD

Also known as acid, LSD was accidentally discovered in 1938 by a chemist looking for a drug to stimulate circulation. Some doctors began researching and prescribing the drug for mental health issues after the war. By the 1960s, LSD – which brings about a 12-hour visionary psychedelic experience – was a potent countercultural symbol.

KETAMINE

Initially a legal anaesthetic first synthesised in 1962, ketamine began to be adopted by club culture in the 1990s, with excessive use known to cause addiction and bladder damage. Since 2019, it's been an FDA-approved depression treatment in the form of Spravato, the first legal billion-dollar psychedelic medicine.

MDMA

Also known as the 'love drug' – or, when in tablet form, ecstasy – MDMA does not produce visuals but delivers empathogenic, heart-opening effects that promote communication. Its use was synonymous with the emergence of rave culture in the 1980s and today it is being considered as a treatment for PTSD.

2C-B

The most notable invention of chemist Sasha Shulgin, 2C-B – also known as 'tripstasy' – delivers an experience that features the euphoria of MDMA and the trippiness of LSD. A popular dancefloor drug and aphrodisiac, it sits somewhere between a stimulant and a classic psychedelic.

How do
psychedelics
work?

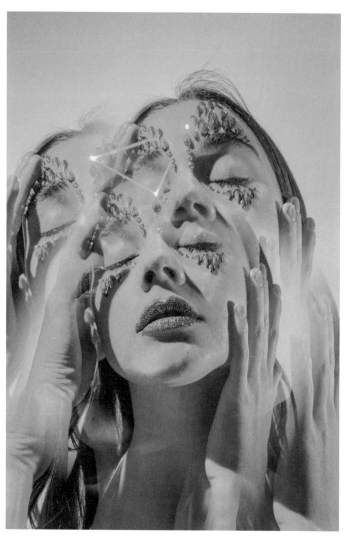

The length and intensity of a psychedelic trip depend on the drug and dosage. A DMT trip might only last 15 minutes, while a large dose of acid can last 14 hours.

What does a trip feel like?

You may already have personal experience of psychedelics – or you may not. Let's begin at the start.

A small dose of magic mushrooms may make colours look more vibrant, and everything might suddenly become strangely hilarious. A bigger dose and your physical surroundings can start to fall away. With your eyes closed, you may feel like you are in a different dimension, seeing kaleidoscopic patterns or even God-like figures that might nudge you towards a mystical experience. For magic mushrooms, trips typically last five hours, but every psychedelic drug works differently (see p.6 for more).

The nature of any psychedelic journey is inherently subjective, but you can expect to feel tingles and rushes through the body and the mind. Moments of clarity might be punctuated by periods of relative confusion. Fears could come up and then be followed by hours of sheer calm and equanimity. Time often becomes irrelevant. Your physical environment may feel like it's expanding or shrinking, or you may feel like you're blending in with it. Simply put, it's a trip. And one to be careful about embarking on.

Set and setting: the factors that make (or break) a trip

The quality of a psychedelic experience is determined by two key elements. 'Set' is short for mind<u>set</u> (one's thoughts, moods and intentions when taking the drug), while 'setting' refers to the physical and social environment where the trip takes place. Two people can take the same amount of LSD in the same place at the same time and have vastly diverging experiences – good trips and bad trips.

The phrase entered the psychedelic lexicon in 1961 when Harvard researcher Timothy Leary said that there is no other greater determinant of the contents of a psychedelic experience than the set and setting – as opposed to the drug itself. Today, it's the reason why medical psychedelic treatment is usually carried out in spaces that feel more like cosy living rooms than intensive care wards. But Indigenous communities have known the importance of set and setting for centuries, guiding ceremonies through singing and drumming to engender a sense of sacredness. The concept of set and setting is believed to have been first theorised in the West by Alfred Hubbard, an LSD-advocate who observed these Indigenous ceremonies in Mexico in the 1950s.

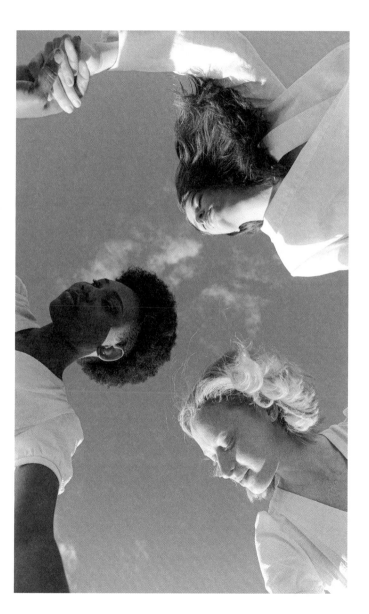

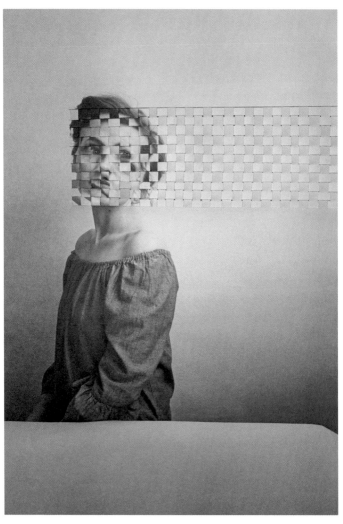

Ego death refers to the complete loss of a person's self-identity. The term was used by Timothy Leary to refer to the first phase of an LSD trip, in which a 'complete transcendence' of the self occurs.
Alma Haser, 'I Always Have to Repeat Myself' (2017).

What actually is ego death?

It sounds pretty alarming. And it can be. Ego death refers to the profound experience of losing the boundary between yourself and the world around you. You might feel like you are melting into your environment or like your feelings have become physical forms that you can see. When people say that tripping made them realise the interconnection of all things, they're referring to this.

Depending on your mindset and existing beliefs, this experience can be hugely liberating – an escape from the burden of everyday existence – or absolutely terrifying, like being hurled into open space. The ego is the part of your mind that gives you your sense of self, and when this dissolves, it can feel as though you're dying – not an experience to take lightly.

Ego death is associated with the concept of enlightenment and unity with God in Zen Buddhism, Sufism and other religions. But complete ego death is rare; most people retain some sense of their subjective self while tripping, so the casual use of the term is often misleading. Nevertheless, the idea points to something deeply transcendental about what psychedelics can offer.

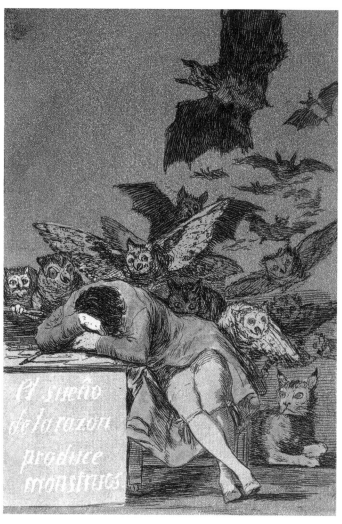

Psychedelics have a very low chance of lethal overdose and are not generally addictive – but that doesn't mean they are without risks.
Francisco Goya, 'The Sleep of Reason Produces
Monsters' plate 43 of Los Caprichos (c.1810).

Are psychedelics dangerous?

You may have heard the phrase 'bad trip' used to describe challenging psychedelic experiences. These might consist of uneasy emotions or disturbing visions, but in some cases, psychedelics can trigger people into crazed states and psychotic breaks.

Since psychedelic use is all about set and setting (p.14), higher doses mixed with lively or chaotic external stimuli can send the mind racing. Some psychologists claim that even bad trips have immense therapeutic value, helping people confront past traumas, though it might be intense at the time. While that may be true, tripping without proper support can have dangerous results, and full-blown psychotic breaks are unlikely to be cathartic. Some never come down, experiencing disconcerting – though rare – after-effects where visual hallucinations can last for months or even years. Some people are even left profoundly destabilised.

Psychedelics may not be inherently dangerous, but their use in certain circumstances is. In 2018, 22-year-old Brandon Begley died at the Soul Quest Ayahuasca Church after he took ayahuasca and kambo (a non-psychedelic frog secretion). He was allowed to drink too much water and had a catastrophic seizure. His death is just one example of several similar cases at psychedelic retreat businesses across the Americas.

What happens in your brain when you take psychedelics?

Classic psychedelics (psilocybin, LSD and mescaline) create a feeling of increased contentment by stimulating serotonin receptors (responsible for the 'happy hormone') in the brain. At the same time, disruption is caused between neural pathways, especially parts involved in remembering. This helps to enhance neuroplasticity – the brain's ability to adapt due to experience. You're generally left more open to new concepts, unblocking ingrained ways of thinking and behaving. It's a moment ripe for alleviating unhealthy states of mind, and you might have thoughts filled with clarity or moments of insight. The apparent neuroplasticity induced by psilocybin can last for weeks, potentially explaining its antidepressant effect.

Imagine your ingrained patterns of behaviour are well-trodden paths. The psychedelic experience is like a fresh snowfall that covers these familiar routes and allows your brain to make new tracks. This is why they can be so effective in changing how we think and behave. It's important to note that there is no *definitive* evidence that proves psychedelics directly enhance neuroplasticity in a long-lasting or straightforward way. Still, countless people insist that psychedelics have fundamentally changed how their brains operate.

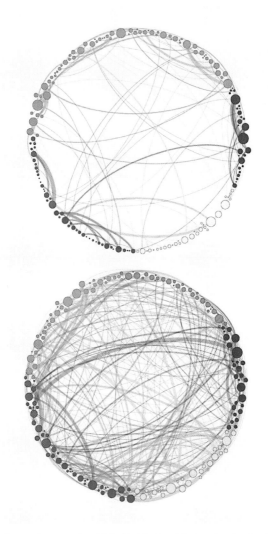

A diagram from a study published by The Royal Society showing the effect of psilocybin on brain connectivity. The top image shows a brain normally; the image below shows the brain under the influence of psilocybin.

How psychedelics impact the default mode network

Psychedelics can alter the brain in profound ways. But how, exactly? Studies suggest that psychedelics disrupt activity in the default mode network (DMN) – a set of brain regions active during introspection and daydreaming.

The science is far from settled, but it seems that psychedelics cause DMN activity to decrease while increasing connectivity between brain regions that don't usually interact. This is perhaps why psychedelics can induce vivid imagery, novel insights and altered perception. Overactivity of the DMN may also contribute to depression and anxiety. By quieting the DMN, psychedelics might help reset dysfunctional patterns of thinking, such as persistent negative ruminations.

'The brain states observed [while on psychedelics] show similarities to deep meditative states, in which increased activity occurs in pathways that do not normally communicate,' psychiatric doctor and ayahuasca researcher Simon Ruffell told *Psychedelics Today*. 'This process has been compared to defragmenting a computer.' In other words, it seems psychedelics can 'reset' the DMN.

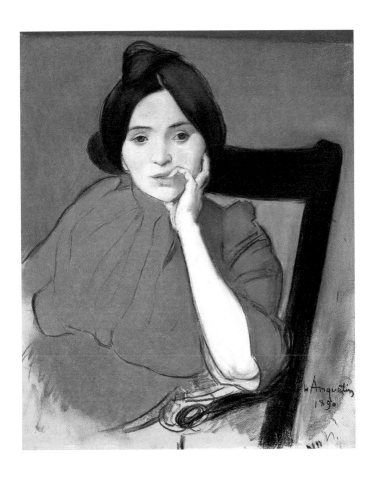

The Default Mode Network is a collection of brain regions that are active when daydreaming. Their activity is decreased through focused meditation – and, it seems, under the influence of psychedelics.
Louis Anquetin, 'Portrait of a Woman' (1890).

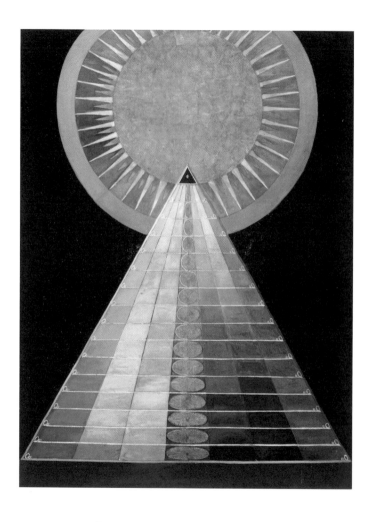

William James first outlined the qualities of mystical
experiences in 1902. Since then, many have used his ideas
as a framework for discussing psychedelic trips.
Hilma af Klint, 'Altarpiece, Group X, Number 1' (1915).

Psychedelics and spirituality, or 'mystical experiences'

Psychedelics have a long history of being used as sacraments and in individual spiritual journeys. In this context, they are often called 'entheogens', a word derived from the Greek *entheos* (divine) and *genesthai* (generate) to describe the spiritual experiences they can induce.

It might seem like psychedelic science and spirituality are gulfs apart, but really, they are two sides of the same coin. The same qualities that make the drugs promising treatments for mental disorders also give them mind-expanding effects, potentially connecting us to higher consciousness or, some say, God. In 1902, psychologist (and nitrous oxide-enthusiast) William James described 'mystical experiences' as being characterised by a sense of unity, a positive mood, a feeling of accessing the divine and difficulty putting the experience into words.

There have been some attempts to study how psychedelics cause these feelings, such as in the 1960s Good Friday Experiment or Rick Strassman's 1991 study on DMT (more on these later). But the intersection between the subjective psychedelic experience and physical biology is underexplored. Some would argue that the very nature of mysticism transcends human understanding.

The origins of
psychedelics

Stoned Ape Theory

Did magic mushroom consumption cause the brains of foraging great apes to evolve? This is the outlandish theory proposed by ethnobotanist Terence McKenna in his landmark 1992 book *Food of the Gods* to explain the mysterious, sudden doubling of the human brain size over 200,000 years ago. The idea has long been ridiculed by mainstream thinkers despite (or perhaps *because* of) some leading figures in the psychedelic world touting the theory.

While the sudden growth in our primate ancestors' brain size is widely accepted, there isn't a scientific consensus for *why* such a neurological leap occurred. According to McKenna, our great ape ancestors may have accidentally eaten magic mushrooms while foraging for food and gained an adaptive advantage. Psilocybin may have catalysed the evolution of cognition that helped homo sapiens develop language, art and religion. Early humans 'ate' their way 'to higher consciousness', bringing them 'out of the animal mind and into the world of articulated speech and imagination,' he wrote.

It's a compelling (and zany) idea, but critics of McKenna's theory point out that there are communities that have consumed magic mushrooms ritualistically for centuries, without appearing to develop any kind of evolutionary advantage over their fellow humans.

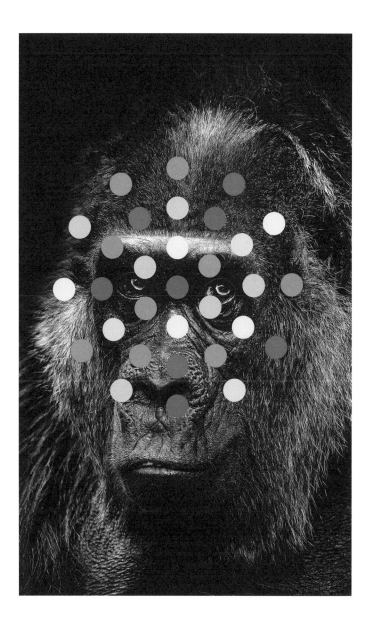

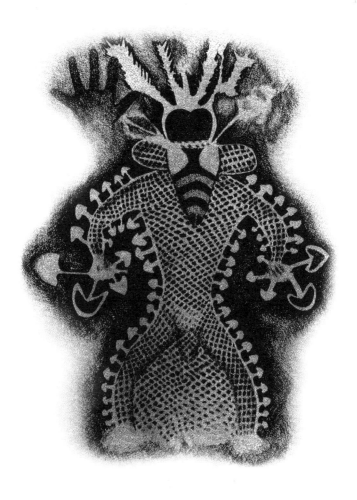

A drawing of the 'mushroom shaman' figure depicted in cave paintings dating back as far as 9,000 years at Tassili n'Ajjer in Algeria. This drawing is taken from Terence McKenna's book, *Food of the Gods*.

How old are psychedelics?

Magic mushrooms date back 65 million years to around when dinosaurs became extinct, according to DNA analysis that can estimate the age of a species.

Plenty of evidence suggests ancient humans took psychedelics as part of spiritual ceremonies and to increase acuity for hunting. Cave paintings at Tassili n'Ajjer in Algeria – some dating back 9,000 years – show shamanic figures holding fistfuls of mushrooms. Effigies made from dried peyote cactus have been found in caves in Texas, and radiocarbon dating suggests they are 6,000 years old – the oldest recorded use of a psychedelic. Archaeologists believe the Texan caves may have been a gathering site for Indigenous Mesoamericans' ceremonial ingestion of the plant. Artefacts found at archaeological sites suggest that the Shipibo-Conibo tribe, who live along the Ucayali River in Peru, appear to have consumed ayahuasca as a sacrament for centuries if not millennia.

In the West, the contemporary psychedelic renaissance – a term referring to the renewed interest in psychedelic medicine and culture since the 1990s – is sometimes framed as remembering ancient practices. But it's important to note that many non-Western communities never stopped consuming such plants. While many in the West are just catching up, the rest of the world never really forgot.

Psychedelics in Africa

Human life began in Africa, and it's likely psychedelic use did, too. Given the rich array of native psychoactive plants that exist on the continent – and probably always have – it would be naive to assume otherwise. Claims to the contrary made by primarily white anthropologists reflect the biases and failures of researchers who have ignored the 'magic plants' used by Indigenous people. The history of ritualistic psychedelic usage in Africa is as rich and storied as anywhere else.

Those doubting anthropologists should try iboga, a powerful Gabonese root bark used in coming-of-age ceremonies featuring autobiographical, all-night visions – also used worldwide as a potent (and successful) addiction therapeutic. The Babongo people, for whom iboga is a sacrament, believe the plant is the mythological tree of life, symbolising a connection between heaven and the underworld.

Other notable African psychedelics include *Boophone disticha*, a visionary – and extremely toxic – plant used by the Zulu tribe; *niando*, said to cause heightened excitement; and *mhlebe*, believed to have prophetic effects. People from the Congo region even have a creation story in which the separation of a divine cosmic mushroom gave birth to existence.

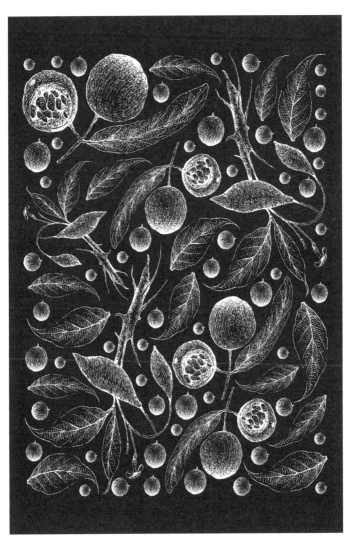

Iboga is a shrub native to Central Africa. Its yellowish root or bark is used in Bwiti spiritual practises, where enormous doses can evoke near-death experiences. Taken in smaller amounts, it has a stimulant effect.

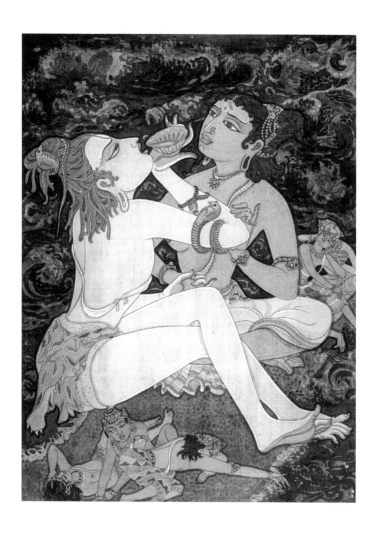

In Hinduism, the Lord Shiva is the foremost drinker of the elusive
soma, enabling him to exist in a constant state of bliss.

Soma, the mysterious Indian psychedelic brew

The Rig Veda – the oldest Hindu holy book, composed in around 1500 BCE – speaks of a mysterious sacrament named soma that can transport its consumer to the realms of the Gods. The writings describe how soma is prepared by extracting juice from a plant, but – seemingly in an esoteric attempt to prevent the uninitiated from accessing the knowledge – fail to identify the sacred, mind-altering substance itself.

Since then, many investigations have given their two cents on its identity: cannabis, fly agaric mushroom, ergot, lotus (which can have a mild psychoactive effect)... the list goes on. There is no extant biological record to draw on, as there are no known traces of soma remaining anywhere, leading some to suggest that the drink is not a substance, but a state of mind, even a deity. 'Soma played a singular role in the Vedic pantheon,' wrote one expert in his search for its identity. 'The poets never tire of stressing soma's sensuous appeal.' Sometimes, the magic is in not knowing.

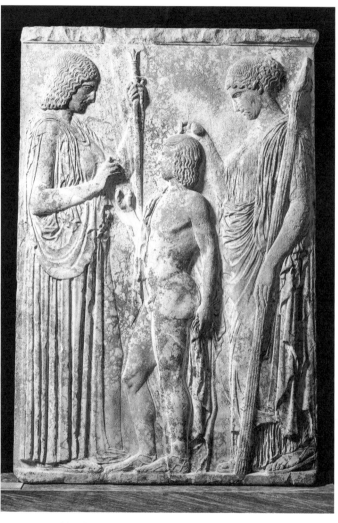

A marble relief depicting the trio of figures central to the Eleusinian
Mysteries: Demeter, goddess of the harvest; Triptolemus, worshipped
as the inventor and patron of agriculture; and Persephone, queen
of the underworld following her abduction by Hades.

The Eleusinian Mysteries

Many assume that spiritual psychedelic usage didn't occur in ancient Europe, but this is a misconception. In Hellenic Greece (323–30 BCE), initiatives at the Temple of Eleusis – a major religious centre at the north end of the Saronic Gulf – appear to have consumed a mind-altering brew called kykeon, made with barley. It was taken after rites involving three days of fasting and dancing, culminating in profound spiritual enlightenment – believed to be a reenactment of the story of Demeter and her daughter Persephone (in which Hades, king of the underworld, abducts Persephone). Some scholars have suggested that the barley used for the drink was infected with ergot, a psychoactive fungus. This would align with the description of initiates experiencing transformational and visionary states, consistent with the effects of ergot alkaloids.

But the rites are not called the Eleusinian Mysteries for nothing: initiatives were forbidden from disclosing the secrets of the rites, punishable with the death penalty if they broke their vow. Although writers like Sophocles, Plutarch and Plato all mention participating, the information they offer about them is scant to non-existent, leaving scholars to speculate about their contents. Whether psychedelics were involved is just one aspect of a mystery we'll never fully unravel.

Food of the gods?
Psychedelics as sacraments

When the Aztecs took mushrooms – also known as *teonancátl*, or 'flesh of the gods' – they would sing and dance beneath the moonlight until sunrise. The mushrooms would be consumed at mountains, lakes and in forests to communicate with the divine and the mystical deities connected to the earth, rain, fertility and agriculture. They were not merely a tool for altered states; they were seen as a medium to commune with the sacred aspects of nature. It's a similar story for the Amazonian communities who use ayahuasca; the peyote-eating cults of the southwestern US and Mexico; and the Bwiti people of Gabon, who utilise iboga as their sacrament.

Most people might immediately associate the word sacrament with the bread shared among congregants in Christian churches every Sunday, but technically, a sacrament can be any consumable that invites inward contemplation and grace – and there is a long history of psychedelics being used in this way.

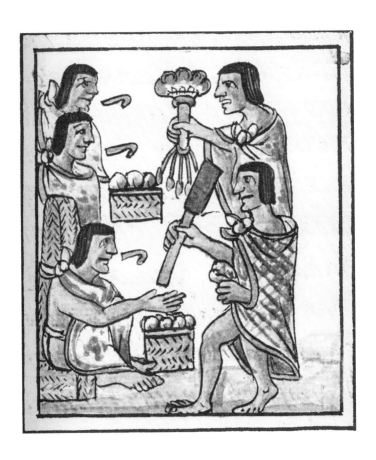

An illustration in the Florentine Codex depicts an Aztec feast in which smiling sacrificial victims consume sacred (psychedelic) mushrooms before their decapitation. The codex was a 16th-century ethnographic study conducted by a Spanish friar.

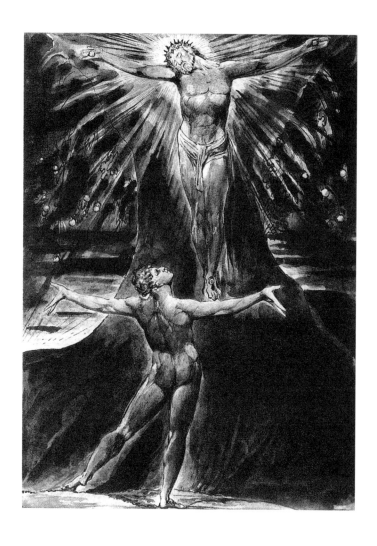

*William Blake, 'Albion Contemplating Jesus
Crucified', from Jerusalem (1804–20).*

The psychedelic roots of organised religion?

Organised religions have historically persecuted psychedelics consumers, perhaps out of fear that they could be used to further personal spiritual journeys and access God without an institutional helping hand. The Catholic church led the charge in the 16th century, with Spanish conquistadors in Peru and Mexico punishing Indigenous communities for whom the drugs were sacred. Yet psychedelics might have more of a foothold in organised religion than we think.

Hebrew University academic Benny Shanon suggests that the prophet Moses received the Ten Commandments from God under the influence of psychoactive plants like those used to create ayahuasca (the vision induced by inhalations from the burning bush). Others have controversially suggested that Christianity was originally a magic mushroom cult. When Jesus is said to have rolled away the stone and resurrected, historian John M. Allegro said his disciples were hallucinating.

Unsurprisingly, these theories have resulted in accusations of heresy and condemnation. But given psychedelics' long history of sacramental usage, it might not be such a radical suggestion. 'The plants are just instruments which induce higher sensitivity, greater insight, spiritual sentiments and creativity,' Shanon told the *Guardian*.

Psychedelics
and the West

William Blake's long psychedelic legacy

In 1765, the painter and poet William Blake, aged eight, had a supernatural vision while walking in a south London park. 'A tree filled with angels, bright angelic wings bespangling every bough like stars,' he recalled. We can assume that the young Blake wasn't on drugs, but insights into reality such as these, which pervaded his work, later inspired Western psychonauts.

'If the doors of perception were cleansed every thing would appear to man as it is, infinite,' he writes in *The Marriage of Heaven and Hell* (1790). 'For man has closed himself up, till he sees all things thro' narrow chinks of his cavern.'

Blake's art featured iconic, otherworldly illustrations depicting nebulous boundaries between realms, divine figures, man and nature. The swirling patterns became associated with 1960s psychedelic poster art, and his writing inspired the countercultural movement, including Aldous Huxley, rock band The Doors and Allen Ginsberg.

While it's possible Blake could have taken magic mushrooms, there's no evidence to suggest this (and recreational usage wasn't common). It's more likely he was born with a brain that, like those with synesthesia, could make connections that the average person can't – unless they take a psychedelic, that is.

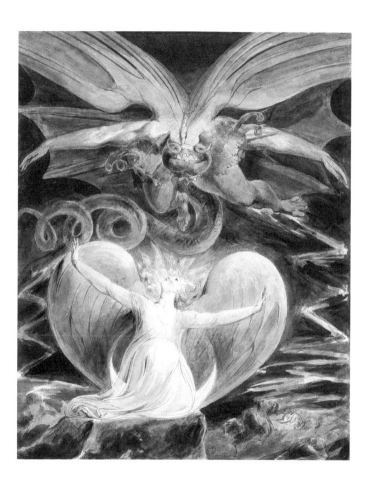

Blake made a series of watercolours depicting
Biblical scenes with fantastical, vivid imagery.
*William Blake, 'The Great Red Dragon and
the Woman Clothed with Sun' (1805).*

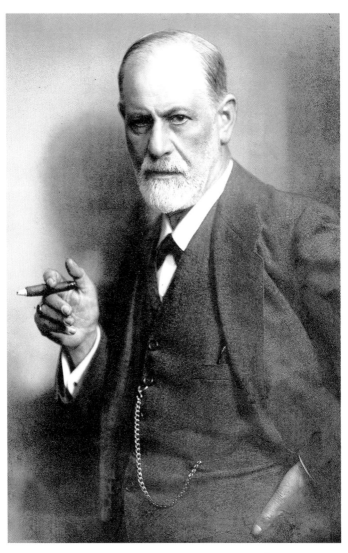

Sigmund Freud was a frequent cocaine user, and wrote his first medical treatise, *Über Coca*, on its extraordinary physiological powers.

Mind-altering drugs in the 19th century

It's often believed that the West encountered psyche-delics in the 1960s, when they were the drugs of choice for tie-dyed hippies, ravers and other anti-establishment folk. But many people in 1800s Europe used then-unregulated mind-altering substances freely (including drugs not typically considered 'psychedelic') – and plenty of well-known intellectuals spoke openly about the positive, enlightening effects of drug use.

Psychologist William James insisted that insights gleaned from inhaling nitrous oxide (also known as laughing gas) were key to his understanding of con-sciousness. Sigmund Freud consumed 'a great deal of cocaine', writing in an 1884 letter to his fiancé that he took it regularly 'against depression and against indigestion'. British chemist Humphry Davy's gigantic quantities of laughing gas propelled him into celebrity, with his vivid accounts of his voyages culminating in the declaration that, 'Nothing exists but thoughts!'

Even Pope Leo XIII enjoyed coca (cocaine-infused) wine – marketed as a restorative medicine. The wine was enormously popular until the prohibition of cocaine and alcohol in the early 1900s. (Incidentally, prohibition forced one maker of coca wine to change his recipe – eventually becoming Coca-Cola.)

Mescaline: the first global psychedelic

Mescaline is the primary psychoactive compound in the peyote cactus, which has been used for millennia in northern Mexico and the southwestern US. In 1897, it went global, opening up new possibilities for research and therapeutic exploration.

German pharmacologist Arthur Heffter was the first person to isolate the drug, ingesting the psychoactive compound to confirm its effects. A series of scientists followed suit, with William James (the 'father of Western psychology'), Silas Weir Mitchell (the 'father of medical neurology') and Havelock Ellis (a controversial, though influential, eugenicist) all giving its visionary effects glowing reviews.

By 1920, mescaline sulphate was available from European pharmacy suppliers as a pure drug. Avant-garde painters like Henri Michaux were soon creating ever more surrealist art under its influence, and philosophers like Jean-Paul Sartre and Walter Benjamin also experimented with mescaline trips. In 1927, German psychiatrist Kurt Beringer published *The Mescaline Inebriation*, a landmark study investigating its effects. A few decades later, Aldous Huxley took it, bringing mescaline into public consciousness with his book, *The Doors of Perception*.

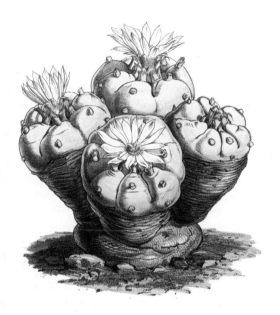

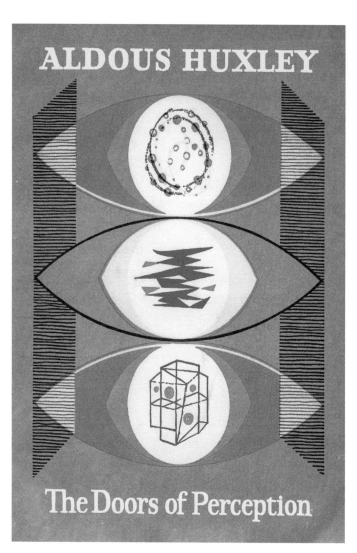

ALDOUS HUXLEY

The Doors of Perception

The first edition cover of *The Doors of Perception*. The
book describes Huxley's experience on mescaline in
1953, culminating in a 'sacramental vision'.

The man who made mescaline mainstream

Man has a limited perception of reality, and taking psychedelics may expand the mind. This was the thesis promulgated by Aldous Huxley, whose experience with mescaline inspired his hugely influential 1954 book, *The Doors of Perception*. 'To be shaken out of the ruts of ordinary perception, to be shown for a few timeless hours, the outer and inner world, not as they appear to an animal obsessed with survival or to a human being obsessed with words and notions,' he wrote. Huxley had been interested in mysticism since the 1930s, learning of mescaline from the research of British psychologist Humphry Osmond. At this point, mescaline was regarded as a research chemical rather than a drug, widely available to buy over-the-counter.

Research around the time had referred to hallucinations (today more accurately called 'visions') as 'distortions' and 'disorders', but Huxley lauded the perceptual changes sparked by mescaline. 'This is how one ought to see, how things really are.' He prescribed mescaline for the happiness of all humankind.

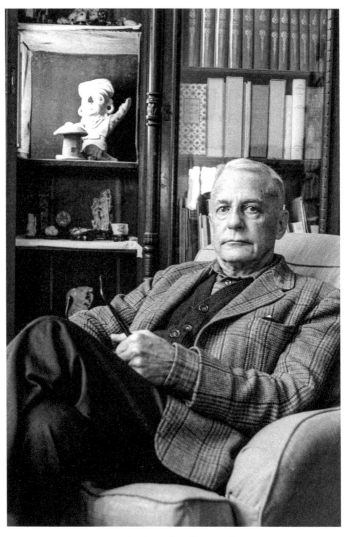

American banker and mushroom-enthusiast
R. Gordon Wasson at home in New York, 1957 – note
the mushroom figurine on the shelf behind him.

The banker whose trip changed the world

In 1955, JP Morgan vice president R. Gordon Wasson (who also happened to be an amateur mycologist) became the first modern Westerner to document an Indigenous mushroom ceremony in a mountain village in the Mexican state of Oaxaca.

Wasson had been searching for a mysterious intoxicating mushroom named *teonanácatl*, chronicled in obscure texts as the 'flesh of the gods' (p.38). His research and enquiries eventually led him to a medicine woman named María Sabina. Wasson broadcast his findings to the world in an article for *Life* magazine, writing, 'We chewed and swallowed these acrid mushrooms, saw visions and emerged awestruck.'

A global tidal flow of magic mushroom discoveries ensued. Outside of Oaxaca, it seemed that relatively few people were eating psychedelic mushrooms on purpose. All that soon changed.

María Sabina and the 'little saints'

When María Sabina performed a mushroom ceremony for Gordon Wasson, she couldn't have known that she was effectively introducing Western society to shrooms (or 'little saints', as she called them). Sabina wasn't mentioned by name in Wasson's original article, but he revealed her identity and location in a subsequent book, against her consent. Mezcal-swigging, LSD-taking, nirvana-seeking American tourists flocked to the town – and directly to Sabina's home – throughout the 1960s, causing social ructions. 'Never [...] were the saint children eaten with such a lack of respect,' Sabina noted. The Western hunger for a shortcut to spiritual enlightenment almost ate the town alive, and Sabina was ostracised, briefly jailed, her property set alight and her son murdered. She died in 1985, aged 91 and impoverished.

Forty years later, her hometown of Huautla de Jiménez not only welcomes the tourism of mushroom-seeking foreign pilgrims, but uses her image to adver-tise it – a cruelly belated vindication of her work. A 20-foot-high official municipal arch is decorated with psychedelic fungi, and a mushroom – figurine or real – is never far away.

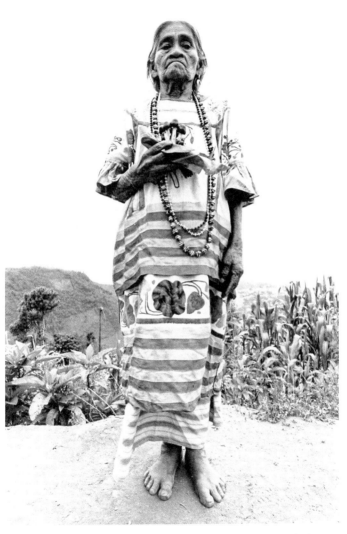

Mazatec wise woman María Sabina. Gusmano Cesaretti photographed
Sabina following a chance encounter with the healer in 1982.

Albert Hofmann's accidental trip

Chemist Albert Hofmann did not intend to create a powerful psychedelic drug; he was trying to develop a respiratory stimulant for the pharmaceutical company Sandoz. He first synthesised LSD (Lysergic acid diethylamide) from an alkaloid found in ergot in 1938 but shelved his discovery until he re-examined the drug five years on, accidentally ingesting a small amount. Curious about the 'dreamlike state' it induced, he took a full dose three days later, on 19 April 1943, and described the results: 'Beginning dizziness, feeling of anxiety, visual distortions, symptoms of paralysis, desire to laugh.'

Somewhat foolishly, he set about on a bicycle ride home, accompanied (thank god) by his lab assistant. 'Kaleidoscopic, fantastic images [...] opening and then closing themselves in circles and spirals, exploding in coloured fountains' ensued. The date has since been immortalised among psychedelics-enthusiasts as Bicycle Day.

Hofmann concluded that the drug could be a useful psychiatric treatment – but not without caution. Hofmann disapproved of the casual, recreational way people took LSD in the 1960s, calling it his 'problem child'. 'I did not choose LSD,' he later said. 'LSD found and called me.'

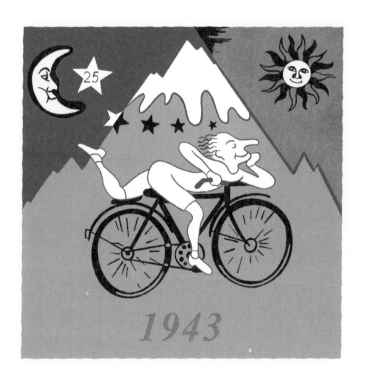

A piece of blotter paper commemorating Albert Hofmann's
accidental discovery of LSD. Blotter paper – saturated
absorbent paper – is a common way of consuming LSD.

PANEL DISCUSSION ON LSD-25.

NURSES LECTURE NUMBER ONE JANUARY 14th 1959 at 8 p.m.
HOLLYWOOD HOSPITAL LOUNGE

Programme

INTRODUCTION// J. Ross MacLean, MD
PANELISTS   A.M. Hubbard, Ph.D. The historical background of
                        hallucinigenic drugs
               U.P. Byrne, MD Practical Evaluation of LSD-25 at
                        the present time.
               D.C. MacDonald, MD Reports on the use of L SD-25
                        in other centres.
               B.L. Skwarok, MD An estimate of the future of LSD-25
                        as a psychiatric aid.

               ROUTINE TREATMENTS AND NURSING STAFF RESPONSIBILITIES
                        AT HOLLYWOOD HOSPITAL
               NURSES LECTURE NUMBER TWO FEBRUARY 11th 1959 at 8 p.m.

                        PROGRAMME
U.P.Byrne, MD   1. Alcoholic Routine A
                   2. Alcoholic Routine B
                   3. Alcoholic aversion Regime

D.C. Macdonald, MD 1. Insulin S ubcoma Therapy
                   2. LSD -25 Procedure
J. Ross MacLean, MD   Nursing staff Responsibilities and general
                      Routine

               THE NEWER MEDICATIONS AND THEIR USES

      NURSES LECTURE NUMBER THREE MARCH 11th, 1959, at 8 p.m.

         Hollywood Hospit,l Lounge

                        Programme

U.P. Byrne, M.D Some of the newer drugs used in Psychiatric Practice

Programme notes from the Hollywood Hospital in Canada, where more
than 6,000 supervised acid trips took place throughout the 1950s and
'60s, investigating the drug as a treatment for addiction and anxiety.

The birth of psychedelic science

After Hofmann took LSD in 1943, psychedelic science was up and running. Hofmann's lab, Sandoz, distributed the drug to researchers around the world, and psychiatrists quickly picked up on its mind-altering effects.

In one Canadian study from 1953 to 1958, LSD was given to around 2,000 people who had failed to give up drinking as part of the Alcoholics Anonymous 12-step protocol. Almost half of them remained sober more than a year later.

Media throughout the 1950s tended to report positively on research into LSD. A 1954 report in *Time* magazine cited experts who said that, as an aid to psychotherapy, it was the best of all drugs yet tested.

From 1963 to 1976, LSD was given to thousands of people at the Spring Grove State Hospital, Maryland (the largest study of psychedelics and psychotherapy to date). The findings corroborated other studies of the period: LSD helps treat mental disorders while relieving pain in terminally ill patients.

This was over 50 years ago. You might think that after such positive results, LSD would be legalised for therapeutic use by now. But you'd be wrong: the road has been anything but smooth.

How the CIA brought LSD to America

It was the early 1950s, and America's fear of communism was at its height. Researching new ways of suppressing their enemies, the CIA became interested in the possibility of mind control and stumbled across LSD. Could the drug be used to brainwash communists into defecting? What if the communists were *already* using LSD to brainwash Americans into changing sides? They became obsessed.

So what did the CIA do to prevent the drug from falling into the hands of their enemies? Naturally, the intelligence agency bought Sandoz's entire supply of LSD for a cool $240,000 (over $4 million in today's money). Spymaster Sidney Gottlieb set up a secret human experimentation programme known as MKUltra. As part of MKUltra, the CIA financed studies into LSD at universities and research centres, hoping to use the data uncovered to their advantage. Ironically, several of the participants in these studies – including beatniks Allen Ginsberg and Ken Kesey – had life-changing trips and went on to extol the virtues of acid, paving the way for the hippie movement.

But the results of MKUltra were far from positive. In addition to backing a handful of legitimate scientific studies, the CIA conducted a decade's worth of deeply unethical experiments with devastating effects.

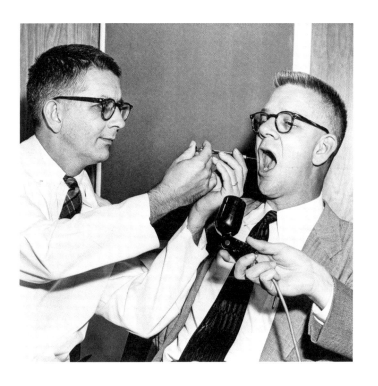

Dr Harry L. Williams squirts LSD from a syringe into the mouth of
Dr Carl Curt Pfeiffer, 1955. Dr Pfeiffer was involved in CIA-funded
experiments researching the effects of LSD on unwitting participants.

The CIA's quest for mind control

Examining the effects of LSD on willing volunteers was one thing, but if the drug was going to work as a brainwashing tool, then the CIA had to test how citizens would react to it *without* knowing what was happening to them. They enlisted the help of Nazi scientists, who had conducted experiments attempting to control prisoners of war at Auschwitz and Dachau, and set about drugging unwitting Americans with LSD over a decade-long period from 1953 to 1964.

In San Francisco, sex workers were paid by the government to bring unsuspecting men to CIA safe houses and serve them acid-laced cocktails while agents observed from behind a two-way mirror. Elsewhere, the CIA drugged asylum patients, prisoners, cops, soldiers and even CIA employees – including Frank Olson, an army chemist who was spiked with LSD and either jumped or was pushed from a 10th-floor hotel window nine days later. Some suggest that more than 5,000 unwitting American servicemen alone were drugged and duped.

Who knows whether the CIA ever did use LSD to interrogate enemy soldiers; records were destroyed in 1973, meaning the full impact of MKUltra may never be uncovered.

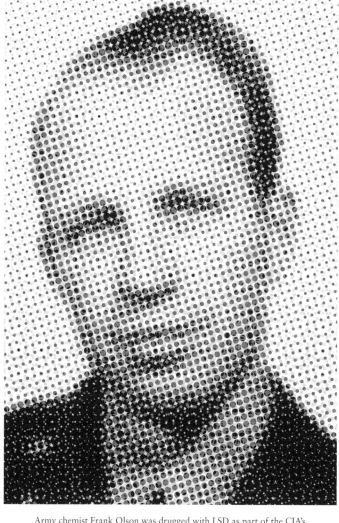

Army chemist Frank Olson was drugged with LSD as part of the CIA's MKUltra programme. It's not known whether his death nine days later was suicide, misadventure or murder, but it is thought that being spiked with LSD could have aggravated Olson's existing mental health conditions.

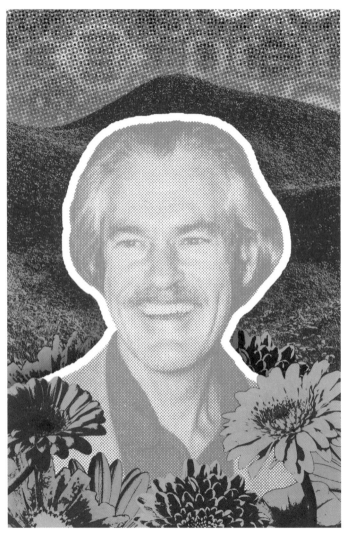

Timothy Leary's influence was far-reaching, inspiring numerous
countercultural figures – not least The Beatles, who wrote 'Tomorrow
Never Knows' and 'Come Together' based on his ideas.

Timothy Leary: Harvard professor turned hippie

He was a strait-laced Harvard psychologist, but after his wife died by suicide in 1955, he was left soul-searching. Five years later, inspired by Aldous Huxley's writings on mescaline (p.51) and Gordon Wasson's article in *Life* magazine (p.53), he tried psychedelic mushrooms in Mexico.

Leary's revealing trip motivated him to found the Harvard Psilocybin Project, in which mushrooms were administered to students as part of the (unauthorised) Good Friday Experiment – more on that overleaf. But he didn't stop there; he continued his campaign to popularise psychedelics, was adopted as a spokesperson for the hippie movement and became famous as the man who ignited one million trips.

Speaking at a hippie gathering in 1967, Leary coined his famous mantra: 'Turn on, tune in, drop out.' The slogan, he later explained, was meant to encourage personal development ('drop out' meaning embrace change), but it was often misinterpreted to mean 'get stoned and abandon all constructive activity'. As the backlash against drugs grew, Leary became increasingly divisive, shunned by the establishment, arrested for cannabis possession (he scaled a wall to escape jail) and dubbed the most dangerous man in America.

The Good Friday Experiment

Do psychedelics really bring us closer to God? On Good Friday in 1962, Timothy Leary and fellow researcher Richard Alpert (later known as Ram Dass) gave psilocybin to ten willing theology students inside the Marsh Chapel, a church on the campus of Boston University. Almost all reported profound religious experiences. Huston Smith, later an author of textbooks on comparative religion, said it was 'the most powerful cosmic homecoming I have ever experienced'.

But Leary and Alpert had not gained institutional approval for the study. Furthermore, their findings didn't mention that one person had to be physically restrained from leaving the church while another was given a tranquiliser to calm down. Criticism of the research mounted, and Leary was dismissed from Harvard the next year.

There have since been attempts to redo the experiment with more rigorous scientific controls. In 2006, half of participants in a Johns Hopkins University study rated their experiences with psilocybin as among their most meaningful spiritual experiences. In 2018, the same university gave more than 20 religious leaders two high-strength psilocybin trips. One participant, Sughra Ahmed, said: 'I now feel a stronger connection to God in everything that I do.' Clearly, Leary and Alpert were onto something.

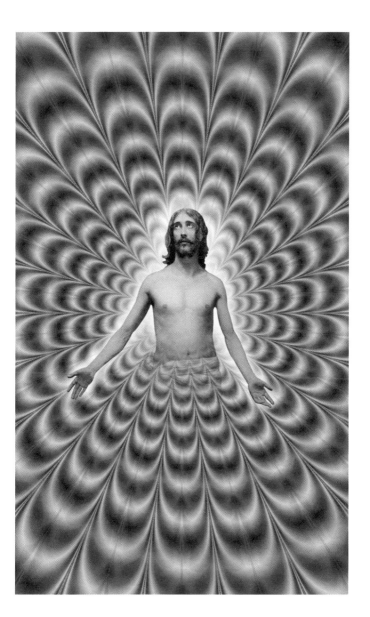

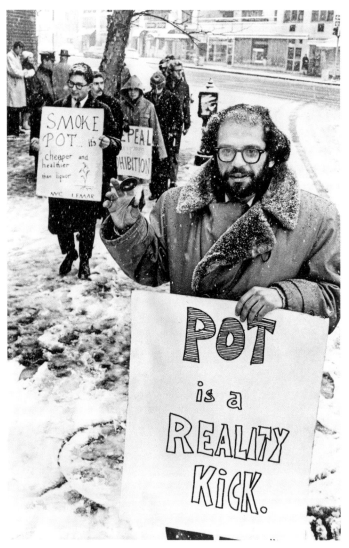

Beat poet Allen Ginsberg leads demonstrators calling for the release of women detained for possession of marijuana, 1965.

The Beat Generation

The Beat Generation was a post-World War II literary subculture that rejected the capitalist status quo and encouraged sexual liberation, drug-taking and free-flowing writing. The term was coined by Jack Kerouac in 1948, appropriating the African American slang 'beat' (meaning 'tired') to describe the emerging underground youth movement. The stereotypical beatnik wore a black turtleneck, hung out in coffee shops and listened to jazz and spoken word poetry. Their bohemian life was powered by amphetamines – until psychedelics came along.

In 1959, Allen Ginsberg took LSD as part of a CIA-financed study at Stanford University (p.60). Meanwhile, William Burroughs was one of the first-ever ayahuasca tourists in the Amazon. He described his experiences in letters to Allen Ginsberg (later published as the highly influential *Yage Letters*). Neal Cassady, along with Ken Kesey, drove a bus of 'Merry Pranksters' across America and extolled the virtues of acid.

As the '50s rolled into the '60s, several Beat Generation figures became central influences of the hippie movement. Ginsberg was at the forefront: 'Everybody who hears my voice, try the chemical LSD at least once,' he said in a 1966 speech.

The hippie movement

The original hippies of the 1960s came hand-in-hand with psychedelic drugs. Evolving from San Francisco's 'hipster' beatniks, hippies protested the Vietnam War, practised free love and took psychedelics as a means of expanding consciousness. In many cases, it was LSD that caused the hippies to question conventional wisdom, become pacifists and give up meat.

The hippie movement began in the late 1950s, gathered momentum with the bus of 'Merry Pranksters' and culminated in 1967 with 100,000 people travelling to hippie epicentre San Francisco (the so-called Summer of Love).

The authorities saw hippies – and the anti-war, anti-establishment message they preached – as a mortal threat to society. Anti-drug propaganda films like *LSD: Insight or Insanity*, in which two cars hurtled into a head-on collision, helped create an image of depraved recklessness. The vignette of acid-taking mania was an unfair characterisation of a hippie movement more interested in euphoric pleasure than psychotic gambits. Still, moral panic ensued.

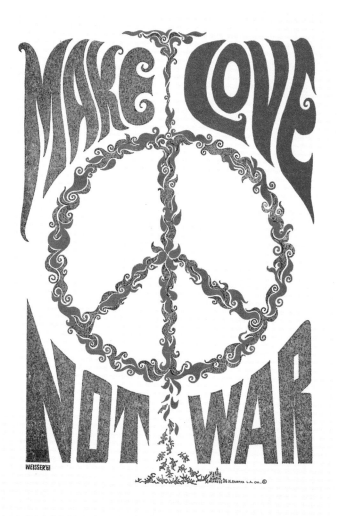

A 1967 poster design by Wilfred Weisser. A globe-trotting hippie originally from Germany, Weisser designed this poster after arriving in San Francisco in the mid-1960s.

Nixon and the War on Drugs

The changing world of the 1960s threatened the status quo. In the US, pacifism and hippie counterculture emerged on a grand scale, protests against the Vietnam War gathered strength and Marxist-Leninist groups like the Black Panthers called for Black liberation. So what did President Richard Nixon do? He declared a War on Drugs, weaponising the view of drugs as fuelling chaos and danger and using this as an excuse to crack down on the protestors and minorities who threatened his Republican programme.

LSD was first in the firing line, followed closely by cannabis. Despite a series of promising preliminary findings (p.59), research into psychedelics was halted, effectively by decree.

It is not a coincidence that this draconian shift happened as the Bureau of Prohibition sought a new war after the federal U-turn on alcohol illegality. A top advisor to Nixon later admitted that 'by getting the public to associate the hippies with marijuana [...] and then criminalising both heavily, we could disrupt those communities [amid a campaign against the anti-war left]. Did we know we were lying about the drugs? Of course we did.' A keen pro-cannabis archive-hunter recently revealed that Nixon even admitted to advisors in 1973 that cannabis was 'not particularly dangerous'.

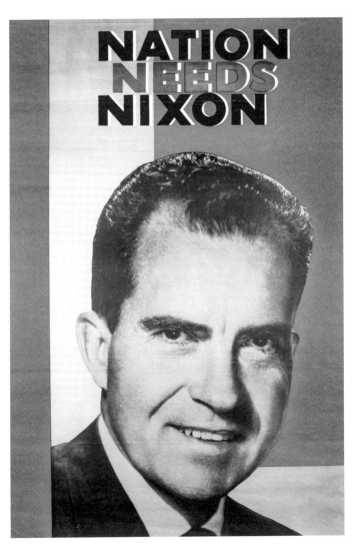

A 1960s presidential campaign poster for Richard Nixon.
Throughout his 1969–1974 presidency, Nixon was
instrumental in pushing psychedelics underground.

Psychedelics go underground

The birth of MDMA

Nixon's crackdown left psychedelic scientists in the dark. Those interested in the drugs' potential had to find new ways of operating, without funding, away from authorities' scrutiny. It was in these circumstances that, in 1977, in a ramshackle home laboratory in California, Alexander 'Sasha' Shulgin synthesised MDMA.

Shulgin was a chemist whose life-changing experiences with mescaline a few years prior had provoked a fascination with psychedelics. After testing MDMA on himself and discovering its empathogenic, love-inducing, non-hallucinogenic results, Shulgin gave it to psychotherapist Leo Zeff, who co-wrote the first scientific paper detailing MDMA's effects on humans.

Under the radar, MDMA surfed from progressive circles in California to East Coast gay nightlife scenes and, by the 1980s, to Europe. MDMA became entwined with club culture, turbocharging ravers and helping to create moments of dancefloor transcendence.

But nothing gold can stay. A 1985 US ban, following claims from officials that the drug was being widely 'abused' across the country, preceded a global prohibition. As a result, scientific research was halted once again. This didn't stop the party, though; it's estimated that more than 20 million people continue to take MDMA globally, making it one of the world's most popular illegal drugs.

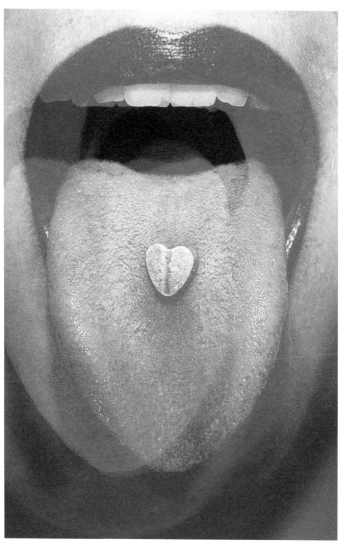

Ecstasy is the street name for pills made predominantly with MDMA, but often cut with other (sometimes harmful) substances to make them cheaper.

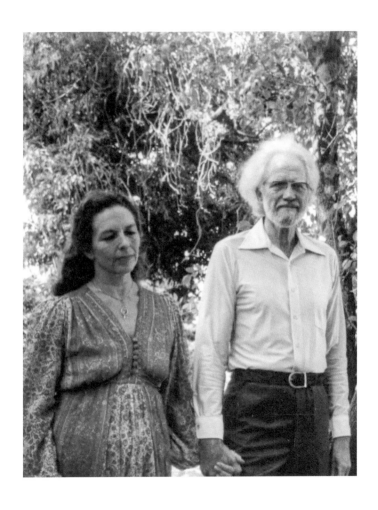

Sasha and Ann Shulgin on their 'spontaneous' wedding day, 1981. Together, the couple were responsible for synthesising over 200 psychedelic compounds.

The couple behind hundreds of psychedelic drugs

In 1978, a year after synthesising MDMA, Sasha Shulgin met Ann. The couple worked together to discover some 200 psychedelic compounds – including 2C-B, a popular psychedelic nicknamed 'tripstasy' for its effects, which are somewhere between LSD and MDMA (p.76). Ann worked as a lay therapist with 2C-B, MDMA and other substances, advocating the use of psychedelics in therapeutic contexts decades before it became fashionable. 'Sasha and I work pretty much as a team,' Ann told the French newspaper *Libération* in 2001. 'We both have the same interests, but our viewpoints are different: he has the scientific viewpoint, and I have the psychological and the spiritual.'

The couple wrote two encyclopaedic books detailing how to create the drugs, publishing the first, *PIHKAL: A Chemical Love Story*, in 1991. This was the final straw for the DEA, who described the texts as 'pretty much cookbooks on how to make illegal drugs'. The Shulgin lab was raided in 1994, forcing Sasha to relinquish his license.

But the cat was out of the bag. The Shulgins continued to work right up until their deaths and left behind a vault containing hundreds more unexamined psychedelic compounds – which researchers are still to this day combing through.

Raving into euphoria

In 1984, at the legendary Starck nightclub in Dallas, Texas, MDMA was sold at the bar. Its patrons would talk about the club's spiritual energy due to the collective euphoria induced by the widely consumed drug. This was before ecstasy – the street name for a pill predominantly made up of MDMA, sometimes cut with other powders – became synonymous with rave culture. Raving itself did not exist yet as such but would emerge in the ecstasy-fuelled acid house parties of Chicago and Detroit at the end of the decade.

MDMA is not a classic psychedelic (technically defined as tryptamines, phenethylamines and ergolines which act similarly on the serotonin system); it's an empathogen, a drug that induces love, empathy, openness and, crucially, makes you want to dance.

It soon made its way to the UK, Holland, Ibiza and elsewhere, where the proliferation of ecstasy on dancefloors was inextricably intertwined with the particular kind of high-octane, transcendental partying that we now know as raving. The year was 1988, and in Britain, this was the Second Summer of Love. This 'bloodless revolution', as music journalist Bill Brewster described in *Mixmag*, 'not only changed how we danced and where, it altered our relationships, our interactions and the way we saw the world'.

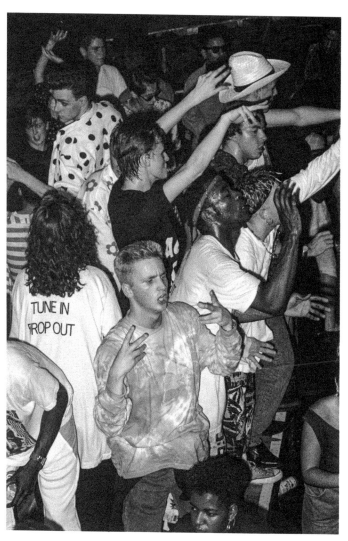

Acid house ravers photographed by Dave Swindells.
One raver sports a T-shirt referencing Timothy Leary's
famous mantra, 'turn on, tune in, drop out'.

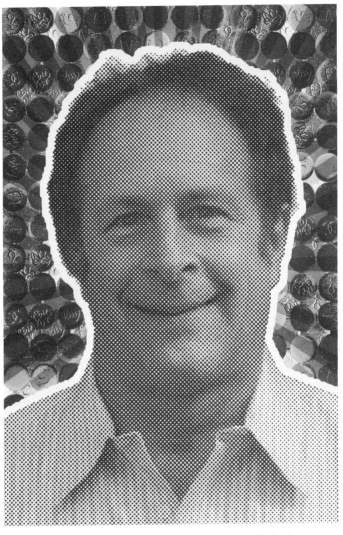

Rick Doblin has dedicated his career to campaigning for legal MDMA therapies, believing that these could revolutionise treatment for those suffering from trauma.

The MDMA crusader:
Rick Doblin

It was 1986 when MDMA evangelist Rick Doblin founded the Multidisciplinary Association for Psychedelic Studies (MAPS) in San Jose, California – the same year that he was awarded a PhD in public policy from Harvard. MAPS was created with the intention of making a legal, not-for-profit medicine out of MDMA, which had been banned the year before.

The task – bringing an illegal drug to the masses – was a tall order, perhaps even a revolutionary aim. MDMA was being attacked by the authorities, who insisted on its potentially life-threatening risks.

Doblin was not to be cowed. Over 37 years, he oversaw MAPS' collaboration with scientists and philanthropists, working to change the public perception of MDMA. 'The key is integrating into society,' he told the *Boston Globe* in 2017, 'to avoid cultural backlash by becoming mainstream, not counterculture'.

Doblin stepped down as MAPS' Executive Director in 2023, a year before federal regulators rejected MDMA-assisted therapy for PTSD patients. But despite that setback, his singular influence and vision for psychedelic medicine has been undeniable. Without Doblin and the advanced-stage studies that he shepherded, MDMA would be nowhere near mainstream medicine.

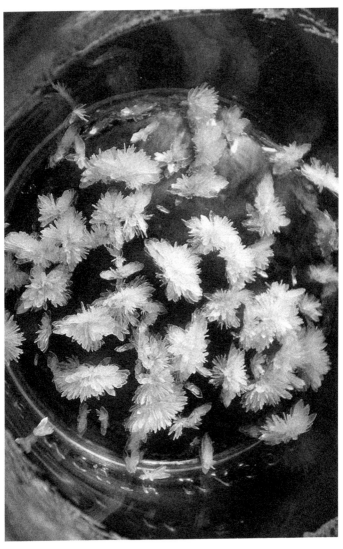

Though naturally occurring in many plants and animals, DMT can also be synthesised in a lab. Pure DMT is usually seen in solid crystal form.

The first government-funded study in 20 years

The period following Nixon's War on Drugs was a difficult time for the study of psychedelics. As professor of psychiatry Dr Rick Strassman wrote in a journal article, 'legitimate human research with hallucinogenic drugs, although of great theoretical and practical interest, involves daunting regulatory hurdles that have discouraged investigators from attempting such work.' But in 1990, after an effective 20-year moratorium on psychedelic research, Strassman managed to jump these hurdles and secure permission for the first-ever clinical study of DMT in humans.

The study involved nearly 60 volunteers who took 400 doses of DMT over five years. More than half of the participants reported encountering otherworldly entities and experiencing deep spiritual insights. Strassman's research culminated in his 2001 book *DMT: The Spirit Molecule*, which included the far-out hypothesis that DMT can be produced in the pineal gland naturally and released into a foetus to 'mark the entrance of the spirit'.

Strassman's research was radical in itself, but more remarkable was the fact it received government support. 'I recognized the importance of my work for the future of American psychedelic studies, and I wanted to make certain that it was performed in broad daylight,' he told *Vice*.

Psychedelics and mental health

The psychedelic renaissance

When journalist Michael Pollan published his 2018 book *How to Change Your Mind*, it became a huge bestseller. The study of 'the new science of psychedelics' captured a zeitgeist. Why were drugs like psilocybin and LSD – which had shown promising medical potential when studied in the 1950s–1970s – still prohibited? Pollan was catapulted onto the speaker circuit and metamorphosed into an elder statesman of psychedelics, ready-made to convince middle America that it was time for a rethink.

Pollan wasn't the first to contest the lengthy ban on psychedelic medicine. Throughout the 1990s and 2000s, researchers and advocates like Sasha and Ann Shulgin (p.79), Rick Doblin (p.83), Rick Strassman (p.85) and Amanda Feilding (p.96) published groundbreaking data on the benefits of tripping. Instead, Pollan's book helped begin a realignment of psychedelics in the popular consciousness as tools for growth and healing rather than countercultural weapons.

'The psychedelic experience is not for everyone, nor should it be,' he wrote. 'It is, however, something that everyone deserves the opportunity to make up their own mind about.'

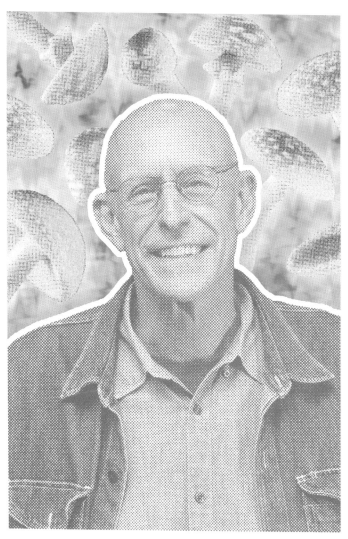

Michael Pollan, author of *How to Change Your Mind* (2018).
Pollan's book is credited with bringing the notion of
psychedelics as tools for healing into the mainstream.

The end of addiction?

This story begins in 1962 with a pair of teenage film students, Howard and Norma. Howard Lotsof, who was dependent on heroin, was experimenting widely with drugs. A chemist friend gave him ibogaine, a psychoactive substance from the root of the iboga plant (p.32). The results were astounding. 'Suddenly, I realised that I was not in heroin withdrawal,' Lotsof later said. 'Where previously I had viewed heroin as a drug which gave me comfort, I now viewed heroin as a drug which emulated death. The very next thought into my mind was, *I prefer life to death*.' He was finally free from the drug's addictive grip on his life.

The inadvertent discovery prompted the couple to dedicate their lives to bringing ibogaine to society at large. Today, there is mounting evidence to suggest that several different psychedelics can be used as treatments for substance abuse, but ibogaine might have the most dramatic and immediate effects. The research is still preliminary, but in one study of people addicted to opioids, six out of 14 people who took ibogaine tested negative for opioids a year later. Ibogaine is already prescribed as a medicine in several countries across the world, including New Zealand, Germany and Gabon (where it is protected).

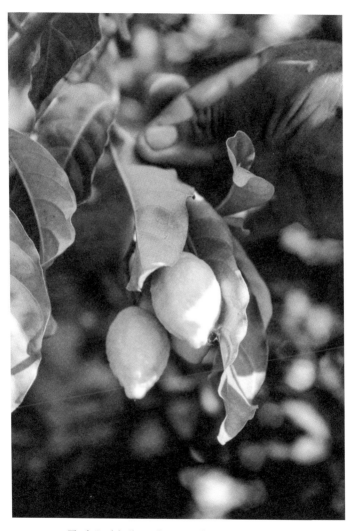

The fruit of the iboga plant varies from yellow to orange,
and can be round and lemon-like in shape, or elongated like
a chilli pepper. Ibogaine is found in the roots of the plant,
which are ground into a fine powder for consumption.

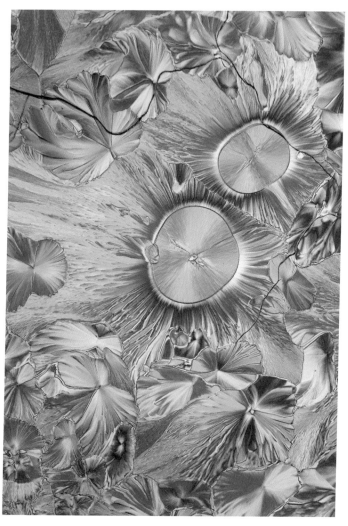

A microscopic image of dopamine crystals. Along with
serotonin, dopamine is one of the brain's 'happy hormones'.
It is thought that psilocybin encourages production of these
hormones, hence its usefulness in treating depression.

How psychedelic drugs may help with depression

In a 2019–2021 study taking place across North America and Europe, 233 people with treatment-resistant depression were given psilocybin combined with therapy. Nearly a third went into rapid remission after a single dose.

The impact this could have on the world is vast: approximately 100 million people globally have stubborn forms of depression. Popularly prescribed medicines like Prozac don't work for everyone, and some patients struggle to come off them.

Aside from a handful of jurisdictions, psilocybin is not currently approved as a treatment for depression, so its legal use is confined to a small number of medical studies. But its results are so positive that some people are sourcing it illegally from wellness retreats.

Depending on the publication of further data due in 2026, the US Food and Drugs Administration may consider approving psilocybin for depression in the coming years. It would mark a jaw-dropping cultural and medical shift if, in the near future, more people were taking mushrooms than pharmaceutical pills.

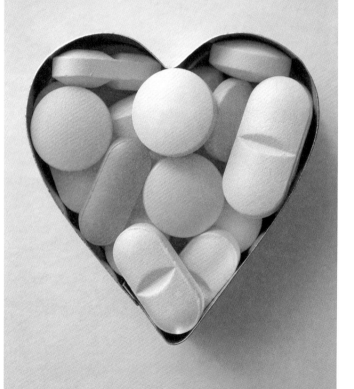

The love drug: psychedelic couples' therapy

Would you take ecstasy to save your marriage? A 1980s study, before the prohibition of MDMA, suggested that the use of the 'love drug' overwhelmingly improves partners' communication with each other. A 2024 paper also suggests psychedelics use leads to better sexual performance.

MDMA-assisted couples counselling is not a legally approved therapy, but increasing numbers of couples are using MDMA informally together. The drug boosts oxytocin, the hormone associated with bonding, and makes it easier to revisit traumatic topics. Shannon Hughes, an associate professor at Colorado State University who co-authored a paper on informal MDMA use among couples, told *Time* that despite MDMA's reputation as a club drug, 'there's this whole subculture of use that's responsible adults with families and kiddos'.

Many couples stay together as a result, reporting stronger bonds and better communication – but for others, taking MDMA can expedite a split. As other-worldly as psychedelics can be, the drugs alone are not going to fix a failed relationship. 'It may be that people are able to reach the natural conclusions of something more quickly,' says psychologist Anne Wagner, 'and hopefully with more kindness.'

Amanda Feilding: aristocrat turned drug policy reformer

She may well be the most influential woman in psychedelic science alive today. Countess Amanda Feilding started experimenting with altered states of consciousness in the 1960s, when she began taking LSD. She later performed trepanation on herself (drilling a hole in the skull, supposedly to improve cerebral circulation). A longtime psychedelics-enthusiast, she founded the Beckley Foundation in 1998 to initiate research into the drugs' impact on mental health and wellbeing. 'Everything I've ever done has started with a personal quest,' she told *The Face*.

The Beckley Foundation has been instrumental in several groundbreaking studies, including producing the world's first images of the human brain on LSD. They have published breakthrough studies investigating psilocybin as a treatment for depression and nicotine addiction – inspired by Feilding herself, who quit smoking after a psychedelic experience. The Foundation advocates for companies to investigate the benefits of microdosing LSD among people with Alzheimer's, and Feilding claims to have observed astonishing initial results. 'I did it to change the world,' she says of her work at Beckley, 'which it has helped to do.'

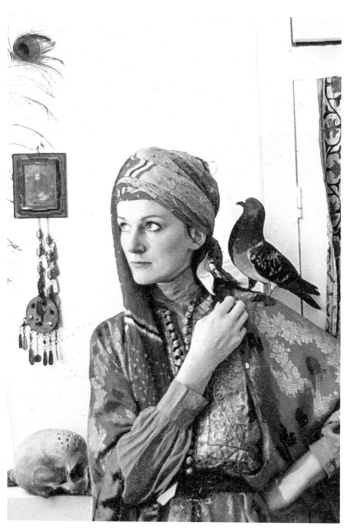

Amanda Feilding, aged 27, pictured post-trepanation. To the left of the image is a trepanned human skull; the practice of drilling holes in the skull to improve cerebral circulation dates from the Stone Age. Also pictured is a tame pigeon that Feilding raised and lived with for 15 years.

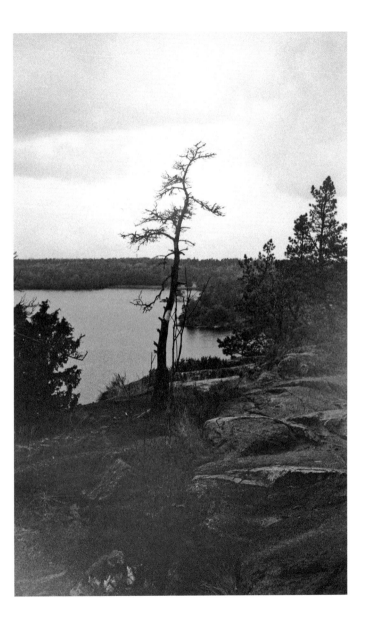

Can psychedelics reduce fear of death?

There is increasing evidence that psychedelics can ease anxiety among end-of-life patients. A 2016 New York University study found that 80 per cent of terminal cancer patients who took a high dose of psilocybin felt less depressed and anxious six months later. As well as reducing fear of death, psychedelics appear to give people a greater lust for life, even from the depths of despair. Anecdotally, several people who planned to undergo medically assisted dying changed their minds after transformative psychedelic experiences.

Thomas Hartle is one such example, inspired to try psilocybin in 2020 after hearing about the study referenced above. 'I didn't have any concept of how life after death could be possible,' Hartle told *Filter*. 'Psilocybin gave me an actual experience of consciousness that did not rely on anything connected with this life.' Hartle eventually died of stage four cancer in 2024.

It's unclear how psychedelics assist people in feeling more serene about their passing. But we know psychedelics can profoundly change our relationship with the world around us. Like in ego-death (p.17), this dissolving of boundaries between ourselves and our environment can be liberating, perhaps leaving people feeling less fearful and more open about what, if anything, comes next.

Oregon, a brave new world

In 2020, voters in the state of Oregon legalised the supervised use of magic mushrooms in a landmark referendum. Now, thousands of people in Oregon have already taken psilocybin mushrooms in specially designated legal centres, with fees ranging from $500 to over $3,500 per trip, plus the costs of subsequent therapy.

The last time mushrooms were legally available in non-research settings was half a century prior. The Pacific Northwest state had to create an entire legal ecosystem from scratch and licence the first legal growers and facilitators, who graduated from approved training programs. A new fungal kingdom was born, and the world is watching: what's happening in Oregon may well be replicated elsewhere.

It hasn't all been plain sailing, though. Since psilocybin remains federally illegal, there are high taxes associated with selling it. One leading facilitator training school has already gone bust, and clinics that aren't backed by big capital have been hamstrung by the costs from the get-go. The regulations don't always make sense, either. Many clients suffer from mental health issues, but the clinics are not permitted to provide psilocybin as a medical 'therapy', requiring users to source accompanying talk therapy themselves elsewhere (something not everyone has the money or inclination to do).

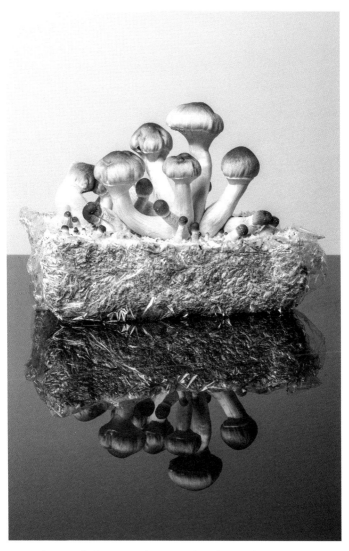

Oregon is the first state in the US not only to decriminalise psilocybin,
but to make it available to the public in specially designed legal centres.

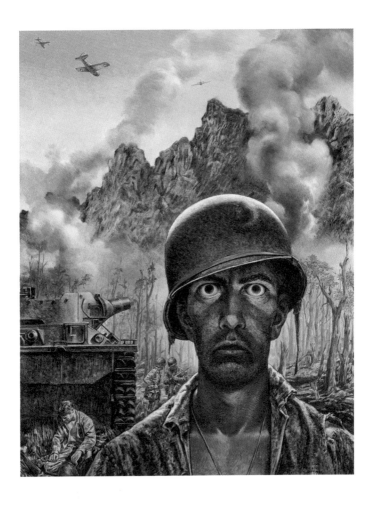

The 'two-thousand yard stare' was a phrase used to
describe the dissociated gaze of soldiers suffering with PTSD.
Thomas C. Lea III, 'That Two-Thousand Yard Stare' (1944).

The bumpy road to an approved PTSD treatment

It is estimated that in the US, on average, more than 15 veterans die by suicide each day. Many of these veterans likely suffer from post-traumatic stress disorder (PTSD), a chronic mental health condition that may be treatable with MDMA therapy.

In two advanced-stage phase trials published in 2021, 71 per cent of patients in the US, Israel and Canada who received doses of MDMA alongside care from a therapist no longer met the criteria for a PTSD diagnosis. The researchers concluded that the findings, which reflected several earlier-stage trials, demonstrated the treatment was a breakthrough therapy with amazing potential. The news was welcomed by military veterans who have been leading campaigns to access the therapy for years.

There were high hopes that MDMA-assisted therapy would be approved by US regulators in 2024, but in a shock ruling, they declined to do so, citing a lack of convincing data – more on this overleaf. The FDA requested further data from a new study, which will take several years, marking a significant setback for the prospect of medical psychedelics.

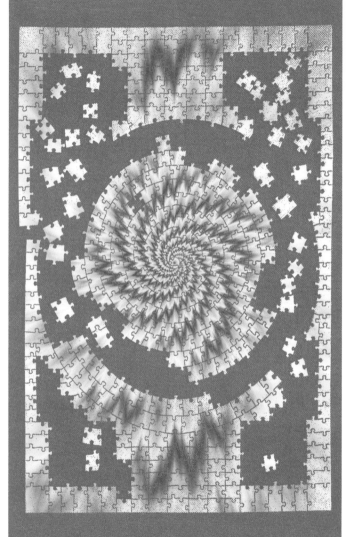

The limitations of psychedelic research

When the FDA turned down MDMA-assisted therapy as a treatment for PTSD, they said there wasn't enough data to approve the drug. After all, the two late-stage trials involved no more than 800 patients, a necessarily small size because the company behind the studies operated solely through donations. As hopes mount about psychedelics' potential, bigger companies will surely get involved, and more funding will enable larger-scale research – but until then, it must be stated that the weight of clinical evidence remains light.

In the 2021 trials of MDMA-assisted therapy for PTSD, 48 per cent of the placebo group also appeared to improve drastically enough to shed their PTSD diagnoses – casting doubt on the study's 'promising' overall results. Equally, a 2024 review of six small clinical trials by the prestigious non-profit Cochrane reported that the certainty of data suggesting psychedelics can treat anxiety, depression and existential distress among end-of-life patients is 'low to very low'. They cited a 'high risk of bias and imprecision' due to small sample sizes.

So, currently, we're stuck in a bit of a psychedelic paradox: big hype, small samples. After all, the data set appears to be a microdose.

When mind expansion meets market expansion

In the West, it typically costs a few hundred million dollars, at an absolute minimum, to bring a new drug to market. Until now, most of the clinical research into psychedelics has been conducted by smaller companies that are more inclined to take risks. But as psychedelic medicine is rolled out commercially in countries like Australia – where psilocybin and MDMA were approved for therapeutic use in 2023 – Big Money (companies wielding financial power) is taking notice. Here is where mind expansion meets market expansion. 'You don't have to be a tie-dye-wearing investor to think of the psychedelic space as interesting,' investor Protik Basu told the *Financial Times*.

What does all this mean for psychedelic medicine? Psychedelics need money to get to the masses. But there are concerns that Big Money, like Big Pharma, does not always have the best interests of patients at heart and may even dilute the psychedelic experience. Stay tuned to see who has the best trip: the patients or the portfolios.

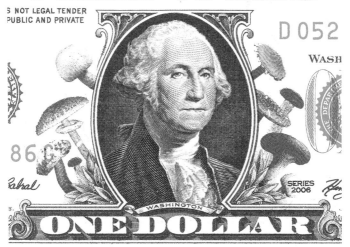

The psychedelic drug market is expected to be valued at a hefty $10 billion by 2028, according to The Business Research Company.

Tripless psychedelics

Despite the potential benefits of using psychedelics to treat mental health issues, many would be understandably hesitant to take a drug that can alter their perception of reality. Could non-hallucinogenic psychedelics – a.k.a *psychoplastogens* or, derogatively, *pseudodelics* – be the answer?

A 2021 study on mice, using a compound similar to ibogaine but without the hallucinogenic effects, reported that it rapidly reduced stress. A paper the year before supposedly 'confirmed' that it is possible to modify a psychedelic compound to produce a safer, non-hallucinogenic variant with the same therapeutic potential. This is good news for those who'd like treatment without a side of intense hallucinations.

There is concern, however, that stripping away the visionary experience might create a blunt tool that only dents the surface of the psyche without unlocking its deeper layers. Experts have argued that the subjective and mystical effects of psychedelics – the reason some people report having the most spiritual moments of their lives – are key to their therapeutic benefits. 'There is a great deal of historical, anecdotal and qualitative data supporting the value of the subjective effects of psychedelics,' researchers from Johns Hopkins University confirmed in 2020.

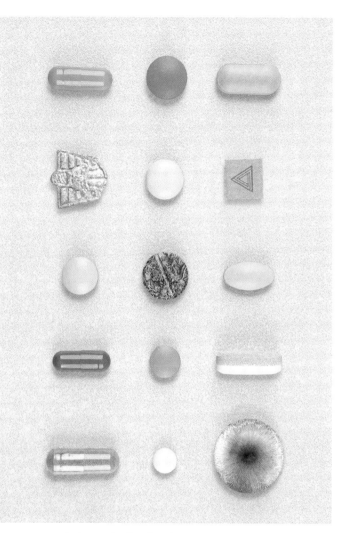

Many who have undertaken clinical psychedelic trips report these as among the most meaningful experiences of their lives, on par with the birth of a first child. On the flip side, trauma from bad trips can be profoundly destabilising, sometimes persisting for years.

Psychedelics
today

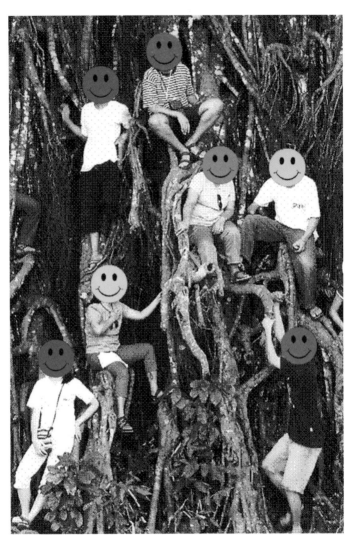

Mushrooms' increase in popularity could be attributed
to how easy they are to find: psychedelic fungi grow
worldwide, often in fields where cattle have grazed.

How popular are psychedelics now?

Some eight million Americans, about three per cent of the population, are estimated to have taken magic mushrooms in 2023. About one per cent of Britons ate shrooms in the same year. While cannabis still outranks all psychedelics in terms of usage, it's safe to say that more people than ever before are tripping – at home, in ceremonies, on dancefloors and even microdosing in the office.

Coming out of the psychedelic closet almost seems in vogue. Coldplay frontman Chris Martin has said mushrooms provided 'the confirmation I needed about how I feel about the universe', Justin Bieber wears a pearly shroom necklace and even Prince Harry attributes mushrooms with helping to process the death of his mother, Diana. *Higher Ground*, a reality TV show aired by one of the leading UK broadcasters, even got its contestants to eat mushrooms as a way of investigating whether a shared psychedelic experience can help people with opposing beliefs find common ground.

So, while mushrooms have replaced LSD as the most popular psychedelic, it shows that hallucinogens are experiencing an unprecedented degree of mainstream buy-in.

Mushroom mania

The growing popularity of magic mushrooms reflects a broader cultural fascination with fungi. In 1997, Dr Suzanne Simard discovered an underground communication network between trees, which she called the Wood Wide Web. Known as the mycorrhizal network, this web relies on the links between fungi and plant roots to share chemical messages. Simard's findings caused ripples in the scientific community, but Merlin Sheldrake's 2020 bestseller *Entangled Life* propelled mycorrhizal networks into the mainstream. 'Fungi embody the most basic principle of ecology: that of the relationships between organisms,' he told *The New York Times*. Interestingly, it was Sheldrake's seminal experiences with psychedelic mushrooms as a teenager that 'startled [him] into curiosity'.

Now, mushrooms – psychedelic and otherwise – are firmly a part of the zeitgeist. Experienced foragers say the number of newbies has increased exponentially, and there have been reported declines in psychedelic fungi as a result (concerned myco-philanthropists on the Pacific Northwest coast have been dumping kilos of wood chips seeded with shroom spores to help spur growth). Meanwhile, construction companies are utilising mycelium to replace polystyrene foam and plastics, and Nasa is growing habitats in space from fungi.

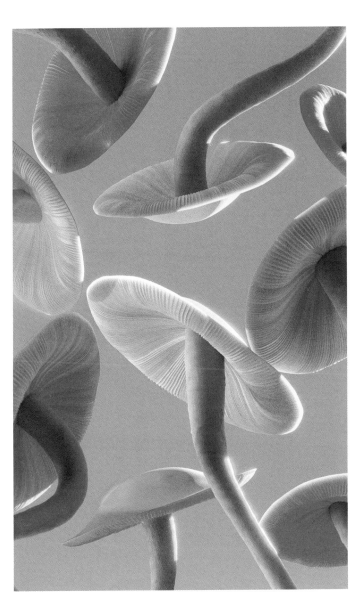

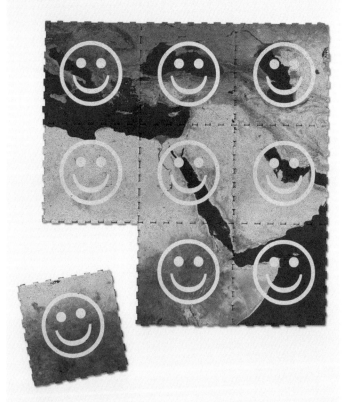

Where are psychedelics legal?

In cities in the US like Oakland, Seattle, Detroit and Washington D.C., plant-based psychedelics are decriminalised (meaning that although they aren't technically legal, law enforcement won't come after you for possessing a small amount). Colorado decriminalised all psychedelics statewide in 2022 and approved a programme of 'healing centres' where you can buy and consume psychedelics under supervision. In Oregon, guided psilocybin journeys are legal (p.100).

This doesn't necessarily mean that psychedelics are about to hit the high streets: there are still strict official guidelines about where and how they can be consumed. But it means that authorities are more likely to turn a blind eye to 'mushroom churches' and other spiritual organisations operating as dispensaries.

In Australia, Canada and New Zealand, certain psychedelics – including MDMA, psilocybin and ibogaine – have been legalised for medical use and can be prescribed by doctors. Psychedelics are also unregulated (meaning, there isn't a legal framework at all) in countries like Mexico, Jamaica, Costa Rica and elsewhere across the Americas, where Indigenous people have long consumed entheogenic plants. Evidently, we seem to be moving in the direction of psychedelic use being more and more permissible.

The magic of microdosing

When it emerged in 2017 that Silicon Valley workers were taking tiny doses of LSD before work, there was a media frenzy. What they discovered is that microdosing can allow you to reap some of the drugs' benefits without any of the uncomfortable or intense side effects. 'It helps me think more creatively and stay focused,' one startup worker told *Wired*. Typically, microdosing involves taking a sub-perceptual dose of the drug (for mushrooms, this would be around 0.1g taken in the morning in capsule form).

Plenty of evangelical anecdotes attest to life becoming better thanks to the daily dose, but backing these up with hard data is tricky. While a lack of evidence doesn't mean the anecdotes aren't true, some people suggest that microdosing is a scam for companies to make more money from selling daily mushroom drops. Some pro-psychedelic detractors of microdosing say people are better off doing a full trip. On the flip side, there are plenty who claim that sub-perceptual and low doses of mushrooms and LSD have enabled them to come off antidepressants and ADHD meds, leaving them happier than ever.

Miracle medicine, or just the placebo effect and self-reporting biases at work? The jury's still out.

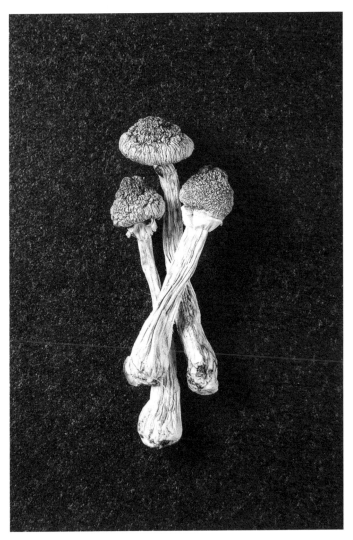

A 2024 study from the University of Maastricht suggested that
not everyone's brain responds in the same way to microdoses,
which may explain the discrepancies in test results.

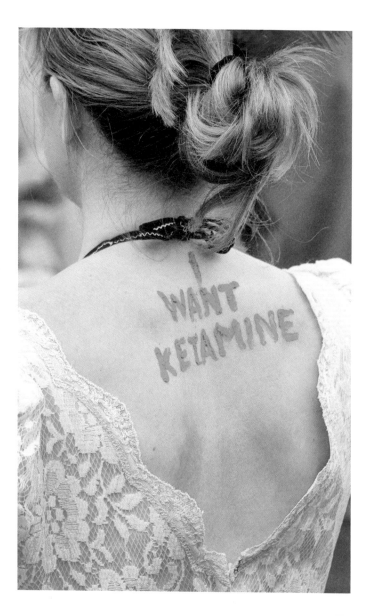

The ketamine boom

Horse tranquiliser, medical anaesthetic, cutting-edge therapy: ketamine has emerged as an unlikely front-runner in the medicalisation of psychedelics due to its comparatively lax classification. Already approved as an anaesthetic, there is far less red tape when it comes to testing it in other medical contexts. The last decade has seen hundreds of ketamine clinics spring up across the US, offering treatment for anxiety, anorexia and addiction with surprising efficacy. Even Elon Musk is a fan, speaking openly about using ketamine to manage his low moods.

In-clinic sessions are expensive (sometimes upwards of $500 for a 20-minute trip), but at-home therapies are a more affordable option, where companies mail slow-releasing ketamine lozenges to patients' homes with pre-recorded trip guide playlists and AI-generated online help services.

At the same time, ketamine has cemented itself as the drug du jour in student halls, on dancefloors and in pop culture. Recreational use has soared – in England and Wales, use has more than doubled since 2016, and in the States, seizures of illicit ketamine grew by 349 per cent between 2017 and 2022. Ketamine is cheaper than other party drugs like MDMA and cocaine – but users build up tolerance quickly, and overuse can have devastating effects on the bladder.

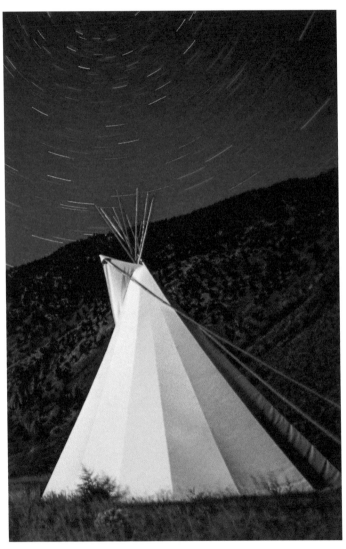

Native American Church ceremonies take place in specially erected tipis. The service includes a fire, singing, prayers and the use of peyote as a sacrament.

The churches where psychedelics are legal

Psychedelics have been used ritualistically for millennia, but over the past 150 years, formalised churches have sprung up, principally in the US and Brazil, where congregants use visionary sacraments as a central part of their worship.

The Native American Church, which incorporates traditional Native American beliefs with aspects of Christianity absorbed from missionaries sent to convert Indigenous peoples, uses peyote to communicate with the Great Spirit (God). The church faced heightened legal issues in 1971 when President Nixon outlawed psychedelics (p.72) but, after years of campaigning, gained a religious exemption for their use of peyote in 1994. A few more have followed suit since then.

But where is the line between sacrament and drug? Commercial entities like retreat businesses can take advantage of the religious freedom laws, offering intense psychedelic experiences to paying customers, who sometimes leave the ceremonies in far worse shape than when they arrived (p.19).

The drug war against traditional healers

When the Spanish conquistadors arrived in Mexico half a millennium ago, they feared that the Indigenous people could harness magical powers by using peyote. Regarded as a portal to God, the colonisers saw the visionary cactus as a threat to their own rule and the Catholic Church. Peyote was banned in a 1620 decree under the premise that consumption of the mescaline-containing cactus was akin to devil worship.

Four hundred years later, people worldwide still face legal repercussions for serving plant medicines. Colombian healer Claudino Perez recently spent two years awaiting trial in Mexico, including prison time, before his case was dismissed. He described the authorities treating him as 'just another criminal [...] They classify us as traffickers.'

The continued persecution of traditional healers is another racist, colonial hangover. And while wisdom keepers are persecuted, the West fetishises and commodifies their cultures through lucrative psychedelic retreat businesses.

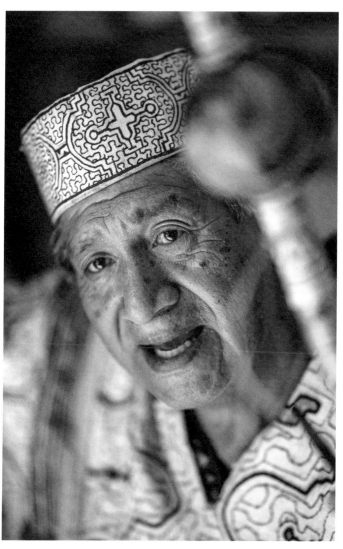

Peruvian shaman Lauro Hinostroza. Hinostroza was arrested in Mexico in 2023 for possessing ayahuasca at a conference for Indigenous medicine.

Toad venom, beer and seafood: psychedelic tourism

Going on a psychedelic retreat is the future of wellness travel among spiritually-minded millennials... as recently reported by *Vogue*. Psychedelic tourism is bringing dollars (and culture clash) to Peru, Gabon, Jamaica, Costa Rica, Mexico and elsewhere. Weeklong retreats, or 'pilgrimages', may include surfing, cacao ceremonies and yoga. Many experience significant healing thanks to their trips, but there have been instances of Westerners becoming paranoid and going on the warpath against their shamans and ceremony participants, even resulting in deaths – as in 2018, when a Canadian man shot and killed an Amazonian medicine woman, and then was lynched as retribution.

As the multimillion-dollar grey market expands, so too do the numbers of shysters and fake shamans. Psychedelic tourism has a dark side. When rapid-acting psychedelics are offered in hotels and on beaches without the requisite preparation and integration, people can destabilise and derealise, with potentially devastating effects. A toad venom trip hosted by a seaside vendor who is also selling beers and ceviche? No thanks.

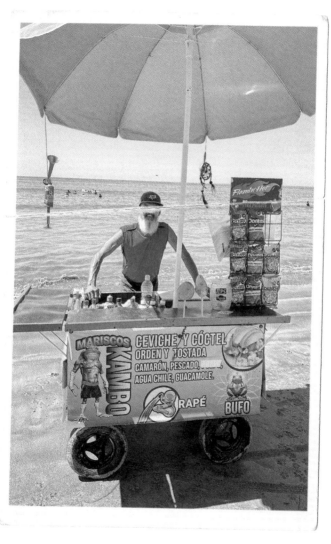

A seaside vendor in Mexico selling bufo (smokeable toad venom) alongside beers and ceviche.

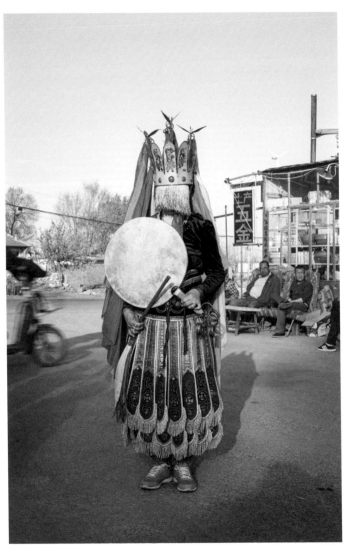

Lilejiluga, a practising shaman in northern China,
photographed by Ken Hermann in 2017.

What is a shaman (and can anyone become one)?

Shamans facilitate psychedelic rituals and communicate with spirits. The term was first used to describe ancient Turk and Mongol religions in the 1600s but was applied indiscriminately by Western anthropologists to describe unrelated Indigenous spiritual practices worldwide. Many of these cultures have their own words for their medicine holders, from the *Mara'akame* for the Wixarika tribe of Mexico (who use peyote as their sacrament) to the *N'ganja* for the Babongo of Gabon, who use iboga.

Traditionally, shamans followed in their parents' footsteps or received callings through serious illnesses (many cultures believe that overcoming serious illness can give you the power to heal others). But the world is now flooded with fake shamans who have paid for 'training' at neo-shamanic schools targeting Westerners. Not only are these schools appropriating the spiritual practices of Indigenous religions the world over, but they often rush people through training programmes in weeks when it should take years, leaving them dangerously ill-equipped for leading ceremonies. With proper training and respect for the cultures you are learning from, shamanism can perhaps be learned. But the title can't be lightly assumed or simply paid for.

A psychedelic future?

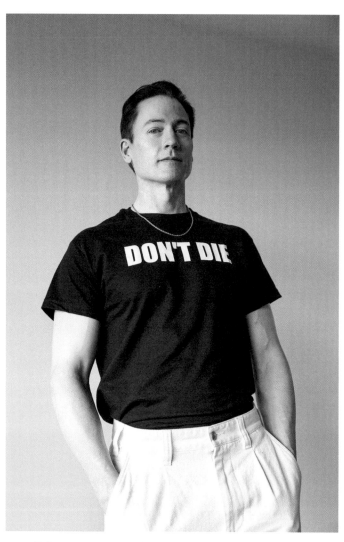

Tech entrepreneur Bryan Johnson sporting his *Don't Die* T-shirt. Don't Die is the name of a programme and online community launched by Johnson with the ambitious aim of 'defeating human death'.

Can psychedelics help you live longer?

Several studies have shown that psychedelics can reduce the fear of death (p.99), but can they actually *extend* life? An emerging subsection of the longevity movement seems to think so.

Tech entrepreneur and longevity guru Bryan Johnson is one such believer, recruiting psychedelics into his bizarre quest for immortality (other things Johnson has done in his efforts to live forever include receiving blood plasma from his teenage son and rejuvenating his penis through electric shock therapy). After advertising his longevity protocol at a 2023 psychedelics conference called Wonderland, Johnson – who has the DMT molecule tattooed on his arm – told the *Guardian*, 'Psychedelics and longevity seem like long-lost best friends.'

But what does the science say? Some early research suggests that psychedelics, when used judiciously, can have an anti-ageing effect on the brain by reducing inflammation. It's also generally accepted that they can help mental health, which in turn reduces stress and enhances cognitive ability, leading to healthier choices. If the connection sounds tenuous, that's because it is; there isn't any hard evidence that taking psychedelics increases your lifespan, though the movements do overlap in a transhumanist vision of the future.

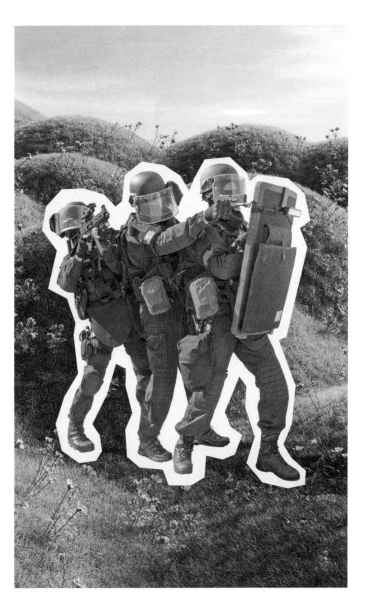

Psychedelics, war and peace

Amphetamines like speed have long been the drug of choice to help soldiers stay alert, but microdoses of psychedelics could offer similar benefits with fewer health risks.

Some soldiers in Ukraine are said to be using ibogaine and ketamine to address traumas swiftly. The US government is also funding research into psychedelic therapy for active-duty soldiers suffering from PTSD and traumatic brain injury. In Israel, one study plans to treat current soldiers with MDMA to prevent complex PTSD from setting in.

Veteran-led campaigns for MDMA therapy have put the spotlight on soldiers' mental wellbeing (p.103) – but historically, similar interventions for active-duty soldiers have had sinister motivations. During World War II, traumatised American soldiers were given a hypnotic pill called Blue 88 that induced a deep, trance-like sleep for two days, then sent back to battle ('a very quick and dirty process,' recalled Captain Ben Kimmelman). It doesn't feel inconceivable that genuine rehabilitation efforts could be exploited to get soldiers back to the battlefield. Indeed, psychedelics commentator Erik Davis has warned that therapy for active-duty soldiers could become 'grease for the military machine'. He has a point: the best way to prevent trauma among soldiers is to avoid war altogether.

A psychedelic (virtual) reality

As if psychedelics weren't wild enough on their own, a recent study saw participants wearing virtual reality headsets while tripping on DMT. Zeus Tipado, a neuroscientist who is leading the research at the University of Maastricht, is hoping to figure out how to 'read' a person's virtual experience using a high-tech brain scanner that can measure perceptual changes and thus help demystify the subjective experience of the trip.

Psychedelic experiments require trips to take place in a reliable setting that minimises the effects of external stimuli, hence why participants are often given eye masks to wear. But VR headsets could offer a way to control the setting even further, coaxing the mind away from vacant thoughts and providing a compelling focus. There are, however, concerns that it could heighten the possibility of derealisation, creating ever greater distance between someone's trip and their everyday reality. Basically, returning to your previous self may become harder.

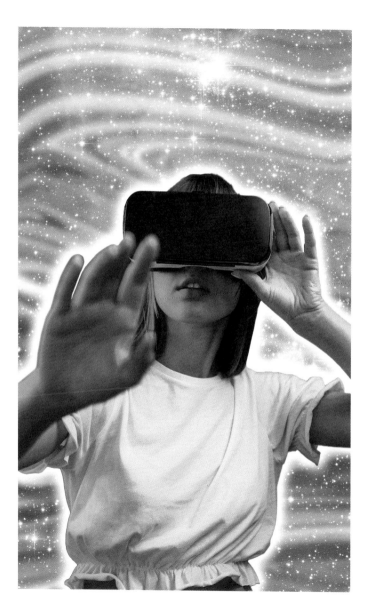

Transhumanism and psychedelics

Transhumanists, many of whom have coalesced around Silicon Valley, believe that the human race might be able to evolve beyond its apparent physical and mental limitations through the means of science, technology… and psychedelics.

Mushrooms and LSD are seen as tools to enhance cognitive function, access higher levels of thinking and open new ways of understanding consciousness, which is central for transhumanists who wish to 'upgrade' the human condition. With the prospect of artificial intelligence exceeding human knowledge on the horizon, some transhumanists and tech pioneers believe that psychedelics might help humans understand consciousness on a deeper level and aid in the development of brain–computer interfaces.

A common critique is that such plans are explicitly anti-democratic and individualist, a means for an already gilded uber-rich class to make even greater profits from disruptive utopian schemes. Still, together they form a weird vision of the future where humans might become more than human, through both technological and psychological evolution.

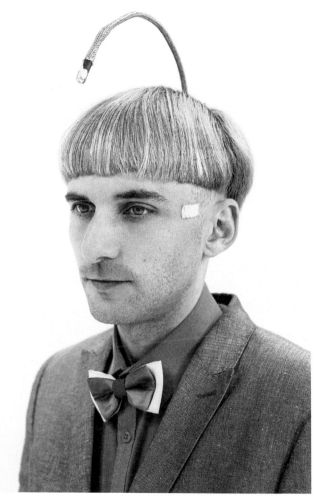

Neil Harbisson, photographed by David Vintiner in 2015. Harbisson was born colourblind, but in 2004 implanted an antenna in his skull that allows him to perceive visible and invisible colours as audible vibrations. Harbisson identifies as both a cyborg and transpecies.

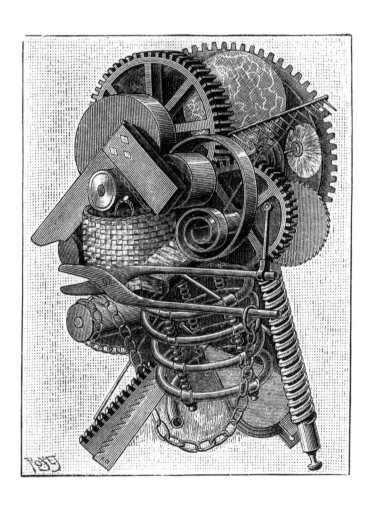

The idea of reaching 'Net Zero Trauma' by 2070 was
proposed by longtime lobbyist for MDMA therapy, Rick Doblin.
William Mason, 'Engraving After the Inventor's Head' (undated).

Is it possible to achieve Net Zero Trauma by 2070?

In June 2023, dressed in a messianic white suit, MAPS founder Rick Doblin (p.83) told a packed Denver auditorium that the mass take-up of MDMA therapy would lay the groundwork for 'net-zero trauma' by 2070. 'I've been working on this since 1972,' he told *The Microdose* newsletter, 'I thought we needed a more challenging vision for the next 50 years.'

The idea is not that no one from 2070 onwards will experience trauma; rather, we'll have the infrastructure in place to deal with it adequately. 'It's kind of just a math question,' Doblin said. 'How many more people are traumatised, and how many did we help get over their traumas?'

The Associated Press dismissed the claim as 'grandiose', but Doblin does seem to have a plan... of sorts. 'We'll need to create therapeutic opportunities for people with lots of trauma and little to no money,' he told the newsletter *Psychedelic Alpha*. 'We'll need to develop group therapy models with local healers to scale the healing potential of MDMA-assisted therapy.'

Ambitious? Certainly. But if MDMA therapy is approved in the coming years, who knows where the road may lead us.

What does the future look like?

The idea of 'Net Zero Trauma by 2070' was met with a mix of hopeful exuberance and scorn – but the heady 'Psychedelic Twenties' may take us to unexpected places.

The rate of US war veterans dying by suicide is typically highlighted as evidence of the need for legal psychedelic therapies as soon as possible. But questions over the affordability of access and the ethical difficulties of war veterans being first in line for treatments have raised eyebrows. Many others have been left traumatised by their psychedelic trips. Meanwhile, as growing numbers of people attest to the transformative therapeutic effects of psychedelics, underground and unregulated dispensaries are popping up all over the place to meet demand.

In the coming years, regulators across the world will consider whether to approve a whole raft of psychedelic drugs, and jurisdictions will continue to decriminalise in the interim. It's fair to say that we're heading for a world where psychedelics are more accessible. Will warnings that mass psychedelic use lead to a more unsettled tomorrow prove true, or will our psychedelic future lead us to calmer, halcyon days? As with any psychedelic experience, the outcome is never entirely certain – but with a world in desperate need of healing, it may be a trip worth taking.

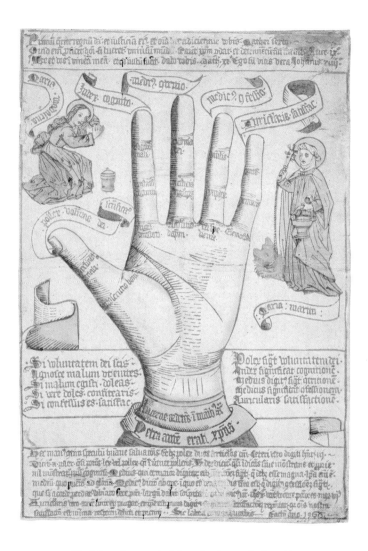

The future of our psychedelic society is yet to be foretold.
'The Hand as the Mirror of Salvation' (1466).